TOWARD A NEW ENRICHMENT... AND FULFILLMENT OF SEXUAL INTIMACY

Love is play; play is love. Both defy death.

Just as children only play with those who are friends, so sexual partners only play with those they love. Love precedes play and follows it. It makes possible the atmosphere of truth, confidence, of festivity, fantasy, and wit that is essential for play to begin. Play, in turn, enhances all these characteristics in a common life together...

To be sexy is to be aware of one's body as an instrument of playfulness, to be able to communicate this awareness to others, and then to commit oneself to a gift of that body in a mutual search for pleasure, variety, and delight. Most people must learn how to be sexy; and to learn how to overcome shame and fear...

This book constitutes a nonfictional statement of the convictions about the meaning of sexuality which animate my novels. The word *meaning* is the key to this book. I am writing neither a sex manual nor a treatise on sexual ethics. Rather I am searching for patterns of meaning by which humans can interpret their sexuality—a task which may be more erotic than a sex manual...

—Andrew M. Greeley

ANDREW M. GREELEY is a distinguished sociologist, journalist, and priest—and one of America's most prolific writers. His bestselling novels include *The Cardinal Sins, Thy Brother's Wife, Ascent Into Hell, Lord of the Dance, Virgin and Martyr, Angels of September, Patience of a Saint,* and *God Game,* as well has his Blackie Ryan mystery series and his second science fiction novel, *Final Planet.* In addition to his novels, he is the author of over one hundred scholarly works and more than fifty nonfiction books, including his highly acclaimed *The Making of the Popes 1978.* Andrew Greeley divides his time between Chicago, where he works as a research associate at the National Opinion Research Center at the University of Chicago, and Tucson, where he holds the post of professor of sociology at the University of Arizona.

NOVELS BY ANDREW M. GREELEY

Death in April
The Cardinal Sins

THE PASSOVER TRILOGY

Thy Brother's Wife
Ascent Into Hell
Lord of the Dance

TIME BETWEEN THE STARS

Virgin and Martyr
Angels of September
Patience of a Saint
Rite of Spring

MYSTERY AND FANTASY

The Magic Cup
The Final Planet
God Game
Happy Are the Meek
Happy Are the Clean of Heart
Happy Are Those Who Thirst for Justice

SEXUAL INTIMACY: LOVE AND PLAY

Andrew M. GREELEY

This book was originally published as two volumes:
Sexual Intimacy and *Love and Play*

WARNER BOOKS

A Warner Communications Company

This book was originally published as two separate volumes entitled *Sexual Intimacy* and *Love and Play*

Warner Books Edition
Sexual Intimacy ©.1973 by The Thomas More Association
Love and Play © 1975 by The Thomas More Association
All rights reserved.
This Warner Books edition is published by arrangement with the author.
Warner Books, Inc., 666 Fifth Avenue, New York, NY 10103

W A Warner Communications Company

Printed in the United States of America
First Warner Books Trade Paperback Printing: February 1988
10 9 8 7 6 5 4 3 2 1

Cover design by David Gatti
Book design: H. Roberts

Library of Congress Cataloging in Publication Data

Greeley, Andrew M., 1928–
  Sexual intimacy.

  Reprint. Originally published as two separate
volumes: Chicago: Thomas More Press, 1973–1975.
  1. Sexual ethics. 2. Sex (Psychology) 3. Marriage.
4. Sexual intercourse. I. Greeley, Andrew M.,
1928–   . Love and play. 1988. II. Title.
III. Title: Sexual intimacy. IV. Title: Love and
play.
HQ31.G78 1988   306.7   87-21633
ISBN 0-446-38556-5 (pbk.) (U.S.A.)
       0-446-38557-3 (pbk.) (Canada)

The instinct of fidelity is perhaps the deepest instinct in the great complex we call sex. Where there is real sex there is the underlying passion for fidelity.
                                          D. H. Lawrence

CONTENTS

INTRODUCTION

In this volume I combine two long essays on the meaning of human sexuality that I have always felt should be in one book. They constitute a nonfictional statement of the convictions about the meaning of sexuality that animate my novels.

The word "meaning" in the last two sentences is the key to this book. I am writing neither a sex manual nor a treatise on sexual ethics. Rather I am searching for patterns of meaning by which humans can interpret their sexuality—a task that may be both more erotic than a sex manual and more challenging than an ethical treatise since the most erotic of human organs is of course the brain.

For most of our history as a reflective species we have been torn by two fundamental interpretations of our sexuality, the "puritan" and the "religious." The former tells us that sexuality is dirty, base, vile, appropriate for locker room sniggers and scatological jokes but evidence that the Creator made an

artistic mistake in ordaining the mechanics of
procreation and the dynamics of the nurturance of
human young. The latter tells us that human fertility
is a hint of divine fertility.

The second position dominated till three thousand years ago: All religions were essentially fertility
cults, a worship of the life-giving power of fertility
and a plea that the fertility, the life, of the crops and
the flocks and the tribe continue.

With the emergence of the world religions, however, and the realization that humans are capable of
transcendence, spirit was imagined to be imprisoned
in flesh, soul constrained by body, wisdom limited by
sexual hungers.

Christianity has been tempted by both interpretations: Because of its Jewish origins and the power of
its own sexual symbols (married sex was considered
to be a sacrament—a revelation—of divine love),
early Christianity, particularly in its pastoral practice with ordinary people, taught that sex was holy.

Catholic Christianity, despite its heavy commitment to the theme of the sacramentality of sex,
broke decisively with puritanism only in the present
era in Pope John Paul II's audience talks on sexuality—
talks that have yet to influence the practice of the
Church or even the Pope's own ethical applications of
his theoretical stand.

Many of the problems of contemporary folk with
their sexuality are the result of puritanism or its
illegitimate offspring, "permissiveness." The churches
didn't introduce puritanism, and we would have a
hard enough time figuring out our sexual needs and
desires if puritanism had never come into existence.
But for much of its history Christianity has not
realized that puritanism is a dangerous enemy. Even
today, as I note in many of the angry letters about

my novels (outnumbered many, many times by the favorable letters), many Christians still think puritanism is official Christian teaching, and not a dangerous heresy. Permissiveness has found an ally in the currently popular behaviorist model of sexuality: Sex is an animal function that need not be subject to religious or moral constraints.

My problem with explicit behaviorists like Masters and Johnson is not primarily theological or philosophical (although I have some difficulties with them in these areas too). My fundamental difference with them comes from my own social science perspective. I am in a remote sort of way a disciple of Max Weber. Hence I am convinced that what distinguishes the human from other animals is his capacity for language. The human develops symbols that enable him to give meaning and interpretation to his behavior. These meanings and interpretations are elaborated into complex cultural systems, and the patterns of behavior that are guided by such meaning systems constitute man's social structure. His interactions with others are relational in the sense that they take place more or less in accordance with the norms and models provided by his culture and social structure and in the sense that he seeks personal meaning in and through his relationships. Human behavior, then, is guided by meaning systems, and human experience is interpreted by these systems. Men and women mate according to the cultural conventions of their society (though not always in precise accordance with such conventions), and they interpret their mating experience by the symbols that their culture provides for them. No other animal acts this way. The scientific observers of human sexual behavior and the wise men who offer advice on this subject (and there are always many such wise men in the marketplace) must take into account man's nature as a culture-producing and a culture-produced creature or they can't know what they are talking about.

Since humans have little in the way of instincts to prescribe what behavior is appropriate, they must fall back on the norms and conventions of the society and culture of which they are a part. These conventions may be more or less functional, more or less appropriate. If they are not subject to review and change as the circumstances in which humans find themselves change, conventions can become rigid and counterproductive. But even if old conventions are swept away (and they rarely are—the more frequent phenomenon is their gradual transformation), the result is not humans without conventions but humans with new conventions.

The behaviorists are surely right when they argue that many of the past cultural conventions on the subject of sex are not pertinent to the post-Freudian, post-Pill society. They are also correct when they suggest that some of the conventions dictated by the traditional wisdom are based on ignorance and superstition. But they are wrong if they think either that conventions can be eliminated from the human condition or that old conventions are easily abandoned. Behaviorism may have to prescind from conventions to do its laboratory research (and the ethics of this prescinding are beyond the scope of the present volume), but men and women cannot prescind from conventions (or "values," to use another word) in their sexual relationships. Books that purport to treat sexuality in a "value-free" context may be amusing, entertaining, titillating; but they will not be of much help to a creature who, whether he wants to or not, cannot help but attach values to his behavior. An authentically value-free book on sexuality (if such be possible) would be of considerable help to a chimpanzee but no help at all to a human.

So there are implicit values in the behaviorist books, and the basic one is that a person can do with his own body whatever he wants to so long as he doesn't hurt anyone else. Such a value may not be a very sophisticated ethical proposition; it is certainly neither terribly new nor very edifying, but it is at least a value. How useful it is depends on how it helps humans to make sense out of the ambiguity and confusions of their sexual behavior. Whether individualistic hedonism is much use as a value may be doubted, I think. The problem with such an implicit value as contained in the currently popular sex books is not that it is wrong, but that the books are not much help. They shed rather little light on complexities and confusions of human behavior. It is, after all, of only small moment to know how fellatio is performed and to be told that there is "nothing wrong" with it when one is always fighting with the wife and finding it difficult to keep hands off the women in the office and feeling plenty guilty about both. Nor do the details of female orgasm help much when one is trying to work up enough nerve to attempt a reconciliation in a love grown sour. It is not that orgasm is uninteresting or unimportant; it is rather that just now it is not especially pertinent.

There is no escaping the fact that the behaviorist approach to sex currently dominates the field. If one arrives at wisdom by counting noses—or the other parts of the anatomy pictured in the behaviorist books—then the value-oriented approach has obviously lost the day. But if one believes that, as John Cobb has put it, "What happens really matters only if it matters ultimately, and it matters ultimately only if it matters everlastingly," then one must dismiss the present behaviorist majority as an unfortunate and shallow historical aberration that is more a reflection on the backwardness of our time than it is on the importance of values in human behavior.

One of the reasons that the allegedly "value-free" approach to sex is so popular is that those who claim to have a "value-oriented" approach have almost universally confused interpretation with morality. In the minds of most people, to have values about sex means to be saddled with a heavy baggage of moral prohibitions. Religion's contribution to sexual behavior is to draw up a list of what ought not to be done; or, more recently, if one is to believe the approach of certain moralists, religion now provides a list of things that in fact it is all right to do despite our feelings of guilt. It remains hard for religionists, either conservative or radical, to understand that religion is not a moral code and that religious interpretation of human behavior has rather little to do with specific prohibitions or permissions. Small wonder that the behaviorists have carried the day, for even if their interpretations are both implicit and shallow, they at least go beyond casuistry.

It is the intent of this book to deal with human sexuality both in the context of the human propensity to seek meaning in behavior and from the viewpoint of a particular religious meaning system—that of a schismatic Jewish sect founded by an obscure Galilean preacher named Jesus. It will not be a morality book; I shall make no judgment on the many current issues of sexual morality that trouble the followers of Jesus, and particularly that branch that in some fashion or other and with greater or lesser enthusiasm professes loyalty to the Bishop of Rome. As I have indicated in another book, I don't think Christianity is especially interested in the morality business; it has other and better things to do, such as providing answers to the most basic questions of meaning that a man can ask. I shall not address myself to questions of birth control or premarital sex but to the question of what light the Christian symbols throw on the ambiguity and confusion that humans experience in their sex lives. The book, then, is not a manual, not a clinical portrait, and surely not a series of answers to questions you always wanted to ask. It is rather an exercise in interpretation based on the assumption that however important clinical information may be—and it is important—it is not nearly so important as interpretation.

SEXUAL INTIMACY:

LOVE AND PLAY

Part One
SEXUAL INTIMACY

1

Let me begin by explicating a number of my basic assumptions:

1. Sexuality in our species is human; that is to say, while it is rooted in the physical and the genital, it permeates the whole personality.

2. All human relationships are sexual; the more intimate they are, the more sexual they become.

3. There is no reason why human intimacy must terminate in genitality, though obviously there is always a radical possibility of this happening.

4. Sexuality is exchange; it is a rhythm of giving and receiving, of taking and being taken, though this rhythm is, of course, not subject to strict economic barter.

5. Marriage is a special kind of sexual intimacy. It is a permanent (or quasi-permanent) genital relationship between a man and a woman. It is the most difficult but also the most rewarding form of intimacy. It is the most difficult because of the physical and psychological complexities involved in such a close relationship between two human beings; it is the most rewarding because there is great physical and psychological pleasure in working out these difficulties.

6. Marriage is both the source and the model of all human friendships. It is the source because the capacity to take and to be taken in the marriage relationship is the most primal of man's social behaviors. It is the model because the love between husband and wife is at least the implicit ideal for all other human friendships. The problems that plague all human relationships are to be found in a special way in marriage; but the joys of all human intimacy are also found in marriage in a special way.

7. I therefore define friendship as an intimate relationship between two human beings in which both become sufficiently open to one another that they are able, at least to some extent, to put aside their fears and suspicions and enjoy the pains and the pleasures of vulnerability. Living with friendship and living with sexuality is essentially the art of living with our capacity for intimacy, with both the demands intimacy makes and the rewards it gives.

8. While friendship is currently the ideal for the marriage relationship, it has not always been so. In the past, many and perhaps most marriages were able to survive in the absence of friendship as I have defined it. Even in the present time many marriages are not in fact friendship relationships. I am not suggesting that in the pre-Freudian era there were few couples who became friends; I say only that society did not hold this up as a critical ideal. The paradox of our own time is that now friendship has become the unquestioned ideal for the marriage relationship, but the human race has not, I think,

developed sufficient abilities at friendship to guarantee that married couples may achieve that ideal.
9. The relationship between friendship and marriage moves in both directions: Not all marriages are friendships and not all friendships are marriages. But friendship is the ideal for marriage, and a married friendship is the model for all human relationships. I speak of friendship and marriage interchangeably, leaving aside the fascinating but highly complex question of the sexual component of human intimacies (across sexual lines or within the same sex) that are not oriented toward genital relationships. (Herbert Richardson's book, *Nun, Witch, Playmate,* has some fascinating observations to make on this subject.) We may take it that since man is a composite of body and spirit, there is no psychic intimacy without some sort of physical intimacy and that there is no physical intimacy, at least not for a long period of time, without a strain toward psychic intimacy.
10. Finally, I assume that the ideal human personality is androgynous; that is to say, it is a personality that has been able to develop both the so-called masculine and the so-called feminine potentialities within it. Given our culture, this means, I take it, that a man can be secure enough in his masculinity to permit the feminine aspects of his personality to emerge, and a woman be secure enough in her femininity to permit the masculine aspects of her personality to emerge. For most people, one must assume, this can only happen in marriage. (Which is not, be it noted, the same thing as saying that in most marriages it does happen.)

With this somewhat lengthy preliminary, let me turn to a number of assertions about friendship:

1. *Friendship is risk taking.* Even the mildest form of human intimacy involves risk, because in intimacy we both take and are taken, we both expose ourselves to the other and reach out to possess the other. If one looks through the long series of activities that constitute the developmental process of a human marriage, we note that it is marked by a number of ventures into that which was previously unknown: dating, courtship, engagement, the marriage event, the development of bodily openness necessary in the genital component of the relationship, the much more difficult development of interpersonal openness for the psychic component of the relationship. Each of these turning points in a developing relationship involves risks, sometimes small ones, sometimes serious risks; and of course the whole process itself is an ongoing risk. Once it ceases to be so, once it has become a relationship that is both complacent and routine, it has lost its capacity for growth and its capacity to maintain the interest and involvement of the partners. Once a marriage, or indeed any friendship, ceases to be a mutual exploration of the complexities of self and other it becomes a bore.

But there is risk in such mutual exploration, for there is risk in taking and being taken. Suppose that one yields to the other and permits him to take one. What, then, if everything is taken? What if there is nothing left? What if one is unable to respond because everything has been given? There is great vulnerability in permitting oneself to be taken. Courage is required throughout the development of any human relationship, and great amounts of it are required at the critical turning points.

And there is equal and perhaps greater vulnerability in taking. What if one reaches out for the other and the other will not respond? What if one attempts to take and the other refuses to be taken? What if one exposes one's need for the other only to be rejected? There is perhaps more risk in taking than in being taken because the taking partner plays the more active role and looks more foolish and ridiculous when he is rejected. Indeed, the fear of appearing ridiculous is one of the more powerful obstacles to human intimacy. I suspect that the reason why so little of the potential of most human marriages, both genital and psychic, is developed is that the fear of having everything taken away or of being made to look ridiculous keeps risk taking at very safe and cautious levels. We all know cases of very attractive human beings who obviously like each other very much and who are so hung up on their fears and insecurities that they are able to move just a trifle beyond mutual psychic frigidity only occasionally. I would argue that such relationships are symbols of most human relationships, in marriage and out. Because we lack the courage to take risks, the courage to give ourselves and to accept the gift of another, we are therefore unable to take advantage of anything more than a tiny fraction of the joys, physical and psychological, that God has intended us to have in this world.

So great is the fear of risk taking that in many relationships there is an adamant refusal to even talk about the relationship. One thinks of the woman who in her desperate need for sexual fulfillment gives a book to her husband for him to read, a book that he resolutely refuses to look at. Or, alternately, one thinks of the vast amounts of time spent in discussion of the clinical details of sexuality without any reference to the primal fears of human inadequacies that are so much more important than clinical details.

It should be obvious that friendship is only possible when passivity and activity are shared more or less equally by both partners of the relationship. One can achieve minimal stability in a relationship in which a division of labor is worked out by which one person does all the taking and the other does all the being taken. But this really represents only an atrophied relationship; in a true friendship, both the taking and the being-taken dimensions of each personality ought to be free to be involved. Many marriages would be much healthier, for example, particularly in the physical but in the psychic aspects too, if the woman felt free to play the aggressive role more frequently and the man the more yielding role. But in our society, a woman can feel free to be sexually aggressive vis-à-vis her husband only when she has been previously assured of her femininity. Similarly, a man, for all the delightful fantasies he may have about what it would be like should his wife become the sexual aggressor, cannot encourage or permit such behavior unless he is reasonably confident of his own masculinity. It is striking that despite the fact that most people have extremely powerful fantasies about the pleasures to be had from breaking out of the bonds of a fixed division of sexual labor, relatively few people escape such bonds.

In both the physical and psychological spheres, then, most human marriages, and indeed most human relationships, do not go much beyond the minimal level that is necessary to keep the relationship from falling apart. The reason for this minimal development is obvious: We are all terribly afraid of risking ourselves in intimacy.

2. *Friendship is rooted in mutual attraction that must grow or it will atrophy.* Social psychologists tell us that the beginnings of all human relationships are marked by two processes. In the first both partners display their wit, charm, intelligence, admirability,

strength. Both are saying to the other in effect, "See how good and great I am. Admire me!" The second process, beginning immediately after the first, is exactly the opposite. "See how little I am. Protect and take care of me. I am strong but available. You should not only be impressed by me, you should also realize that I need you." This almost simultaneous plea for admiration and care involves a simultaneous manifestation of greatness and littleness, of strength and availability. Good friends become quite skilled in manifesting to the other both strength and weakness, greatness and littleness, admirability and need. They come almost to the point of overwhelming each other with power and strength, but stop short only to collapse (literally or figuratively, depending on the relationship) into each other's arms for comfort and support. The rhythm of appealing and impressing is a subtle one, just as is the parallel rhythm of taking and being taken. It is essential that both partners participate in both sorts of activities, but it is also essential that they become sophisticated in adjusting to each other's cues. Each partner fits the rhythm of his own behavior into that of the other, neither yielding his own needs completely to the relationship nor permitting his needs to dominate the relationship. A friendship is like a free-floating modern dance or a subtle jazz combo; the rhythm is always continuous and always somewhat similar, yet never quite the same. The partners know how to adjust to the other's cues and simultaneously provide the other with appropriate cues.

It is important to emphasize that this free-floating rhythm never becomes static, not at least if it is still alive. In any relationship where both partners have become confident that their adjustment problem has been solved, it is safe to say that there is little left of the relationship. When adjustment ceases, the relationship has become dull; the music has stopped; the dance has ground to a halt.) Unfortunately, many people grow weary of the dance and tired of the music (Certainty, stability, and fixed, predictable patterns seem much more satisfactory than the exciting but wearing process of continuous innovation. It is time, they say, that we settle down. We have taken enough risks. It is time to be sensible now. But when a human relationship settles down it has lost its vigor and its drive. Fear, uncertainty, and insecurity have triumphed over excitement, challenge, and ingenuity.)

3. *Friendship is an alternation between hiding and revelation, between keeping secrets and telling them, between mystery and blatancy.* Friendship is self-revelation and exploration; but the revelation is never complete and the exploration is never finished. There are times when we are complete mysteries to the other, and there are other times when we seem obvious and transparent. If we were mysterious all the time or blatant all the time, the other would quickly lose interest. The merely mysterious person is inaccessible, and the merely blatant person has no subtlety or complexity.

In all human relationships we begin as strangers and slowly discard the protections and veils, the masks and the defenses behind which we have been hiding. But we need help from the other if we are to reveal ourselves both because we need his assurance that self-revelation is safe and because it is a delight to have him share the act by which we reveal ourselves. The delight will be transient, however, if we believe that once the veil has been dropped there will be no more mystery left in our personalities. It is the promise of friendship that at no point will there be an end of new discoveries. The goal, then, is not to reveal the total self all at once, for this is impossible; it is rather to reveal the self in such a way that the other knows ever more about us while his appetite is whetted to know more. As we drop the masks and veils of defense (a process that reveals our self not only to the other but to us too), we must insist that the other permit us to share as recipient and active agent in his own self-revelation.)The mutual psychological stripping process is unlike the physical stripping, which is certainly appropriate and essential in any marriage friendship. Psychological self-revelation is not a series of discrete events following more or less the same pattern with a definite beginning and a definite end; it is rather an ongoing process that once begun must go on constantly, never to end, at least as long as the friendship lasts.

It follows, I think, that there must be grace and elegance in the process of self-disclosure. There is a naive kind of pop psychology, popular especially with immature people who have no toleration for either complexity or ambiguity, in which it seems necessary to learn all about the other as soon as possible on the grounds that once self-revelation is complete the relationship can really begin. One finds this crude, brutal approach to self-disclosure in certain encounter groups where the fundamental assumption seems to be that if one tells everything immediately, intimacy will be automatically assured.

But, in fact, self-revelation is not something that can be completed before friendship can begin. It is an essential component of friendship for as long as it survives. Intimacy must be developed slowly, gradually, elegantly, with the proper combination of mystery and blatancy, of caution and risk. It cannot be forced crudely, directly, roughly. It is part of the natural rhythm of friendship that there are times when we disclose to the other more than is expected and other times when we offer less than is expected. We stimulate the other's desire to know more about us yet hold back until the right time for revelation has been reached. Too much self-revelation too soon would overwhelm and repel; too little would bore. We tell enough about ourselves to keep the other interested, to make him want to come back to learn more, to encourage him; but we also wish to indicate that there is always more to be learned, that there are always new delights to be revealed on another day.

It has often seemed to me that one of the functions of fashion has always been to combine mystery with blatancy at the most obvious physical level— self-disclosure with the promise of far greater things to be revealed. The old morals books used to rant against this, but I think from our present perspective we can see that fashion—obviously within some limits of taste—plays an extremely important part in the rhythm of human relationships. Beachwear is a marvelous symbol of both mystery and blatancy. The muumuu reveals practically nothing; the bikini, practically everything. In the interaction of the two we can see the process of self-revelation neatly symbolized.

Style, grace, elegance in self-hiding and self-disclosure must continue at every stage of a relationship. When there is only blatancy, or only mystery, there is trouble. In marriage or in any human friendship in which there is nothing more to be revealed, no new delights to be discovered, no new tricks to be displayed, no new fun to be enjoyed, there is no vitality. Whoever our friend is we are always in the process of attracting and she or he is always in the process of attracting us. Simultaneously, of course, we are revealing ourselves because the friend demands to know more, and is revealing herself or himself to us because we are demanding to know more. Self-revelation, then, is not merely an active disclosure; it is a response to a demand for disclosure. We encourage the other to demand that we reveal more of ourselves, and then reveal it in response to that demand. We withhold ourselves, yet we lead the other to insist on learning more, and we are perfectly delighted to share our mysteries. We are afraid to probe into the depths of the friend's mystery, yet we find such probing powerfully attractive as the friend leads us down to them. The dance goes on, then, until one or both partners lose their nerve and the rhythm is broken. Whatever rationale is offered for breaking the rhythm, the real reason is always that one and usually both persons have decided to call things to a halt; it is too risky, too dangerous to go on.

4. *Friendship is a rhythm of conquest and surrender.* In a healthy friendship, we never completely conquer the other nor do we ever completely surrender. Once the conquest has become complete, once the surrender is over, the relationship becomes routine and monotonous. If we are absolutely sure that we possess the other, there is nothing left for us to do. We must be convinced that it is still necessary for us to work at conquering, and yet all the time have sufficient signs that our work will be successful. Simultaneously, we must demand of the other that she or he work seriously at continuing their conquest of us, while at the same time communicate to the friend that we are delighted by the efforts and that the work will be successful.

One breaks out of the bonds of loneliness, fear, and isolation by offering oneself; but the act of offering is also an act of pursuit. To make oneself available for taking is to aggressively pursue taking. We must be confident of our own attractiveness to offer ourselves. We must be convinced that we have something minimally worth taking, and we must also be confident of our own strength and power to take. We want the other for ourself, but we also want to belong to her or him. There are deep and powerful fears in our personalities that say that being conquered and conquering is not worth the effort; if it were, we would probably fail anyway. Intimacy is painful. Two human beings brush up against one another in close psychic quarters and, inevitably, conflict, friction, difficulty, and misunderstanding appear. It is not worth breaking through the barriers of the other's hostility and defensiveness. We would only be jumped if we tried. Nor is there any point in attempting to attract the other to us because he or she does not like us in the first place, and how could anyone like us? It is physically difficult for two people to live in close quarters. It is even more difficult psychologically. We want to be left alone; we want privacy; we want the lonely but safe little segment of isolation we have built for ourselves. Conquest and surrender are romantic dreams that have nothing to do with the harsh nature of the real world.

Intimacy, then, is always difficult, and when it stops being difficult it stops being intimacy. It is not easy to know which strategy is most appropriate. Is it time now to break through the other's defense with vigor and force and possess fully? Or is it time to break through defenses by subterfuge? Or do we want the other to tear aside our defense mechanisms? And how do we persuade—indeed, seduce— the other to do so? These questions are not easily answered. Much less is there any answer that is always right. Routine, certainty, simplicity, established patterns simply are not possible in so complex and intricate a relationship as friendship.

The imagery that I have used in previous paragraphs has obvious physical implications, but I would insist that since man is spirit, psyche permeating body, the language is even more pertinent when one describes the far more difficult challenge of psychic conquest and surrender. We use imagery with physical overtones because it is the only imagery we have available, but physical conquest and physical surrender are relatively simple biological exercises—at least if we wish to make them so. Virtually anyone can engage in them with a greater or lesser degree of skill. Psychic conquest and psychic surrender are much more difficult, and by no means is everyone capable of them.

Now, it may well be said that all of this is very interesting, or perhaps not so interesting, but what has it to do with theology? What does it tell us about divorce, remarriage, birth control, extra- or premarital sex? My answer is, probably nothing. I am not at all sure that it is the function of Christian theology to comment on many of these things. We probably have something pertinent to say about indissolubility, reproduction, the importance of human life, respect for the human body; but I think these are secondary considerations in a theology of sexuality. That we think them to be primary is a sign of how narrowly constrained are the perspectives of our own time. The really pertinent question to ask is, what light does the Christian symbol system throw on the anxieties, the fears, and the ambiguities involved in human intimacy? This is a question that I think ought to be placed not at the end of any theology of sexuality but at its very beginning.

What I have been engaged in thus far is an

exercise in Paul Tillich's theological method of correlation. One describes as best one can the ambiguities of a given human experience, and then one asks how Christian symbols illumine that experience. I have insisted that the fundamental ambiguity in marriage, friendship, and sexuality has nothing to do with divorce, birth control, or homosexuality. The real ambiguity is rooted in man's pathetic desire for unity with others and his abiding fear of unity, of his passionate delight in his own vulnerability combined with his terror of being vulnerable, in his profound enjoyment of the sweetness of being able to trust and his bitter response to the possibility of having his trust betrayed. In other words, man desperately wants friendship and love, but he is terribly afraid of taking the traumatic risk of self-exposure that is necessary for love. Shame, a conviction of his own worthlessness and unlovability, tells man that the risk is not worth taking and that even if he should take it, he would be betrayed. Can the Christian symbol system make any response to this primal fear of rejection?

The act of giving oneself in friendship, and particularly the act of giving oneself in a permanent genital relationship, involves the basic core of one's personality and the basic conviction one has about the nature of Reality, with a capital R. If Reality is benign or gracious, then it is ultimately safe to take and be taken because no matter what happens, a gracious Reality will protect one. If, on the other hand, Reality is malign, capricious, arbitrary, then love is a risky business and surrender bound to end in disaster. Most men hesitate somewhere between Macbeth's comment that life is a tale told by an idiot, full of sound and fury, signifying nothing and Father Teilhard's comment that there is something afoot in the universe, something that looks like gestation and birth. Hesitating as they do between a belief in graciousness and a belief in capriciousness or malignity, they can give themselves in friendship and love only partway. I would argue that he who is a Christian, that is to say, one who is fully committed with his total personality to the revelation of God as contained in his words through Jesus Christ, does not hesitate; he is on the side of Father Teilhard's interpretation. While the thought of conquest and surrender may strike terror in his heart, the terror is not strong enough to stop him. I am not saying that only the Christian is capable of friendship; but I will say that a convinced, committed Christian has a far better motivation, a far deeper rationale for friendship than anyone else. The Christian knows that the Really Real is gracious.

More than gracious. One of the most important questions to which any religious system must provide the answer is, do we consider the Really Real to be accessible? Does Reality, or God, or the Gods, care about us? Can we deal with the Real? Must we appease it, must we plead with it, must we remonstrate with it, must we remind it? The Christian symbol system assures us that the Real is accessible, and it goes far beyond that when it tells us that the Ground of Being, the Ultimate, whatever we want to call it, is too accessible by far. Our God is not patiently standing by and waiting for us to offer love; he is actively and vigorously pursuing us. Our God, as I have pointed out in my book *The Jesus Myth*, is presented to us as one who is madly in love with us. Old Yahweh wheeling and dealing in the desert, the father running down the trail to embrace the prodigal son even before he can speak his act of contrition, the mad farmer showering a full day's wage on men who hadn't even worked, Jesus forgiving the sinful woman before she even spoke her sorrow, the crazy shepherd leaving a whole flock of sheep to go find one lost, foolish one, the nutty woman searching the whole day long for a tiny coin lost in the straw floor of a Palestinian hut—these are all symbols of a God whose love for us is so strong that, by human standards at least, he would be said to be mad. Our God is a God who for some crazy reason wants to be friends with us. He wants not merely to take us for his own (an absurd concept, surely); he also wants us to take him for our own. He is a God pathetically eager to reveal himself to us, a God who is quite ready to surrender himself to us, a God who in both the Old and New Testaments delighted in revealing himself as a lover hungering for the body of his bride.

The Christian symbols, then, say it is all right to love. "But, surely," you say, "there is nothing new or startling in that. It is scarcely a relevant revelation. Everyone knows that it is all right to love."

If everyone knows it, how come so few people do it?

Our relationships are characterized by stored-up resentments, awkward divisions of labor, frustrated dreams, vast areas that by mutual consent are never discussed, trade-offs by which certain defense mechanisms of both partners are inviolable, subtle aggressions and manipulations, and brave pretenses to the outside world that all is well between us.

This is the love by which all men shall know that we are followers of Jesus?

The revelation of Jesus tells us that we can move beyond such stalemates and break out of the rigidities that keep our joys and pleasures at such a low level. I think most of us understand implicitly that this is the message of Jesus, but we do not want to believe it because if we do, a profound revolution in our lives will have to occur. We will have to transform ourselves (or "repent" as the scripture used to translate the word *metanein*). And no one wants to do that.

Much better that we argue about celibacy, birth control, abortion, infallibility, Norman Mailer, Germaine Greer—all the really important issues.

If we reject the Christian imagery of God, let us reject it for the right reasons. Let us dismiss it because it is absurd or blasphemous or too good to be true or disgraceful or embarrassing. Let us not reject it because of papal infallibility or birth control or *Humanae Vitae* or clerical celibacy or pop versions of Sigmund Freud or clichés quoted from the counterculture and self-proclaimed radicals. Father Schillebeeckx has said that Christianity is the revelation that humanity is possible. I would go further and say that Christianity is the revelation that friendship and love are possible, that we are free to love, that man need not be afraid to give himself over to friendship, to take and be taken. For if the Really Real, the Absolute Ground of Being, *ipsum esse*, proclaims itself as a friend, then the whole universe is out to do us good. The joys of human friendship turn out merely to be an anticipation of the great life of friendship and joy prepared for us by this spendid, dizzying, crazy God of ours, whose Word made flesh manifested himself to us in these incredible words: "Behold, I do not call you servants; I call you friends."

2

In a certain Catholic parish not so long ago a layman was given the opportunity of preaching the Sunday homily. (I daresay no one consulted the other laity as to whether they wanted to hear a lay preacher at all much less this particular one.) A clinical psychologist and (heaven save us) a marriage counselor, this layman devoted part of his "homily" to quoting statistics that proved *(a)* there was no evidence that premarital intercourse had any negative effect on marriage adjustment, and *(b)* there was no evidence to support the frequently heard contention that those who failed in their first marriages were very likely to fail in their second. For some unaccountable reason the parishioners who heard this "homily" were more than a little offended by it.

Leaving aside the question of whether it is in good taste for Catholic scholars to use the Sunday pulpit as a means of shocking the laity who are not as sophisticated as they, there remains the question of whether the empirical data the psychologist quoted have any real pertinence to the discussion of values for sexuality in marriage.

Much of his data, I think, would be greeted with raised eyebrows by professional researchers, who would want to know where the study was done, who did it, what kinds of questions were asked, and, especially, what kind of sample was involved. (In many articles purporting to provide information about the "sexual revolution," it turns out that the data are based on research done in college counseling clinics—scarcely a random sample of the American people.) One might also wonder about the theoretical assumptions underlying his presentation. Anyone who has paid much attention to the literature on marriage adjustment knows that the strongest predictor—frequently about the only one that matters—of marital adjustment is whether the two parties grew up in a family where the relationship between husband and wife was basically healthy and happy. If the man and woman are from such families the odds on a satisfactory marriage adjustment of their own are very high. On the other hand, if both of them are from relatively unsatisfactory family backgrounds, it can be reasonably expected that they will have a very difficult time working out a satisfactory relationship. Premarital sexuality may very well be an "intervening" variable between family background and marriage adjustment. It may indicate a childish or exploitive approach to sex that one learned in one's family of origin and will practice in one's own family. It is the immaturity of the exploitiveness that will disrupt the marriage and not the premarital intercourse, which may or may not have been a sign of immaturity and exploitiveness.

But most important of all, one does not arrive at

sexual values by counting noses. Even if it turned out
that every remarriage after divorce led to a very high
level of marital satisfaction, this finding by itself
would say nothing about the desirability of divorce;
nor would a strong positive relationship between
premarital intercourse and marriage adjustment settle the question of the morality of premarital intercourse. I will yield to no man in my respect for the
ability of survey research to provide useful and important information for decision making, but survey
research is no solution to moral and ethical questions. Ultimately our values depend neither on what
everyone does nor on rather narrow statistical measures of whether something "works" or not but on
our view of the nature of man and of human relationships. Empirical research certainly provides
input for information on our ethical wisdom (another name for our views of the nature of man and
his relationships), but anyone who works profes-
sionally with the tools of survey research knows
how inadequate they are even to address the fundamentally empirical problems that are their legitimate area. As the principal norm for ethical
wisdom, survey research is about as appropriate as
first-grade arithmetic would be for dealing with
astrophysics.

But there is an implicit assumption in much of
the popular and semiserious literature that attempts
to derive a sexual ethics from the Kinsey report or
its more sophisticated successors, and that assumption is the strange notion that "modern man" is the
only intelligent and enlightened people that ever
lived. We are the first members of the human species
who have been sexually "liberated," at least in any
considerable numbers. Everything that was said in
the matter of human sexuality before Jung and Freud

is irrelevant. There is nothing to be learned from the past, and our only appropriate stance vis-à-vis the wisdom of the past on human sexuality is to liberate ourselves from its rigid superstitious norms and from the guilt feelings that those norms impose. Our predecessors were ignorant, unenlightened, uninformed, stupid. There is nothing to be learned from them; we can only learn from our own contemporaries. Therefore, we take surveys to find out what our contemporaries are doing and decide that whatever the majority are doing is moral. If only we can free ourselves completely from the nagging scruples that say that maybe, just maybe, there is something to be said for the old prohibitions, we would become sexually free and all our "hang-ups" would disappear.

I fear that this "temporal ethnocentrism" is widespread, particularly in the half-educated segment of our population, that is, the segment that thinks the shallow half-truths served up in the college lecture room or counseling center really represent wisdom. It is terribly difficult to discuss sexuality with this substantial component of the American population and not run up against the stone wall of the assumption that we are enlightened about sex and our narrow, rigid, prohibitive ancestors were not.

I am not attempting to defend the traditional sexual wisdom; it certainly had its limitations and inadequacies. Much less am I prepared to defend the rigid norms that attempted to specify this wisdom for concrete situations (but frequently in fact distorted it). The legalism of the moral theology books, the catechisms, the confessional—and the legalism of primitive tribal codes in non-Christian cultures, for that matter—is rarely an adequate expression of ethical wisdom, though the human race even today is hard put to make do without codes. But what I do insist on is that the norms of the past deserve to be understood on their own terms and from "the inside." The casual dismissal of traditional wisdom with cheap arguments (such as "the only reason for indissolubility is to provide care for the children") or bad statistics is not a sign of enlightenment but rather of superficiality and immaturity. Thus, as a social scientist analyzing the nature of human relationships and of human friendship—as described in the last chapter—I am convinced that there is a strain toward permanence in human relationships. I therefore think it is stupid to refuse to examine the almost universal human wisdom on the subject of the permanency of the marriage relationship to discover whether it may possibly speak to some aspects of the human condition that we arrogant and supremely self-confident moderns may have missed. Mind you, to say that there is a "strain toward permanence" in sexual relationships does not necessarily commit one to the present requirements of the code of canon law, but one should examine the possibility that the code is trying to cope, however ineptly and inadequately, with what is a very real human dilemma.

This is not a book about indissolubility, birth control, abortion, homosexuality, extramarital intercourse, transvestism, spouse swapping, or bestiality, and I do not propose to be sidetracked into a discussion of any of these essentially peripheral issues. But I do wish to assert that those who equate traditional human wisdom with specific answers on these questions merely display their own lack of wisdom and sophistication.

The most fundamental insight that primitive

man had about sexuality is one that we frequently overlook or forget: that it is a raw, primal, basic power over which we have only very limited control. Primitive man invariably viewed sexuality as sacred, because for him the "sacred" was the "powerful," and sexuality was one of the fundamental forces that kept the universe going. We have "prettied up" sexuality with thousands of years of civilized conventions and now we have rationalized it by the use of glib psychotherapeutic terminology, hence deceiving ourselves into thinking calm, cool, casual discussion is a meaningful and effective way of coping with our sexual drives. Ancient man knew better.

The most ancient human works of art that we have discovered are figurines unearthed from the ruins of human communities that existed in Siberia thirty thousand years ago. They are simultaneously sexual and religious. Primitive man knew his life depended on the fertility of the fields and of animals, that if the crops failed or the herds did not reproduce he would die. He also knew the continuation of his tribe depended on human fertility. Since fertility and life were so closely connected and since life was something sacred, fertility was sacred too. But ancient man also knew what tremendous power his own sexuality had over his own behavior. He was afraid of that power because he knew that it could drive him into a frenzy. He did not understand it, he could not contain it, and therefore, like every other power that was both strong and mysterious, his own sexuality became something sacred.

The incredible variety of sexual taboos that primitive man devised represented an attempt, frequently misguided and occasionally bizarre, to contain that raw, primal force so that it would not disrupt the fragile relationships that bound him together with the other members of his village or his clan. Modern man may dismiss human concern about sexuality as "guilt hang-ups" and he may argue that sex can be "casual," but in fact the only reason some modern men can practice what they think is casual sex is that society has built up elaborate structures of conventionality that enable it to more or less effectively prevent untamed sexuality from tearing it apart. What is called "casual" sex really isn't casual at all. It involves the violation of some sexual conventions within the protective context created by other sexual conventions. One need only see the movie *A Clockwork Orange* to know what human society would be like if a sufficiently large number of its members decided to practice really casual sex. The result would be anarchy, with the fabric of society coming apart as more and more of us took possession of any readily available sexual partner.

Our ancestors may not have understood many things about sexuality (it is just possible that there are many things that we don't understand either). Their conventions may have been ill-advised, counter-productive, and harmful to the individual person; furthermore, many of the conventions may have deteriorated into hard, rigid legalisms that no longer serve the function for which they came into being, but at least they understood what many of us apparently do not: The rational, casual, "chatty" approach to sexuality is simply inadequate to cope with such a raw, basic human hunger. In the absence of strong conventions, untamed sexuality will destroy human society. The ancients knew this; we apparently do not know it. In this respect, they were much wiser than we are.

And yet every one of us experiences his own sexuality as imperious and demanding. Our craving for sexual satisfaction, for sexual relief, for sexual union permeates our being and frequently dominates our behavior to the exclusion of all else. One man put it to me quite simply: "When I am traveling, if my wife isn't with me I end up either chasing waitresses or punching bartenders." Those who delight in the rational, casual vocabulary of Dr. Ruth will be offended by such a blunt, earthy description of the sexual drive. They will forget, or try to forget, that their own sexual hunger has frequently led them, if not exactly to chase waitresses or punch bartenders, to come close to very similar behavior. Our sexual hunger frequently tells us to do things that appall our more rational and civilized personality dimensions. Our hunger for sexual satisfaction is probably not as powerful as our hunger for food, but then few of us in contemporary America are hungry for food for long periods of time. We are able to cope with that hunger by eating three times a day. Satisfaction of our sexual appetites is not nearly so easily accomplished.

Because our sexual hunger is so powerful and so pervasive, it becomes involved with every strange and bizarre trait in our personalities. There is not a single neurotic defense mechanism that we've developed that is not at least partially sexual in origin and partially sexual in its manifestations. Our defense mechanisms exist to protect our own fears of sexual inadequacy; and we impose neurotic behavior on others as a form of sexual aggression, which substitutes, though just barely, for more obvious and more explicit sexuality. Even the most mature of us (and who is all that mature?) has severe problems preventing his sexual hunger from disrupting his life and destroying his values. Sexuality is a raw elemental force that sweeps us along like a thirty-five-mile-an-hour wind would toss a tiny sailboat on the waters of Lake Michigan. Any approach to understanding and living with sexuality that does not take into account the immense and undifferentiated power of sexual passion is naive and self-defeating. The body of a sexual partner, only remotely available—fully clad in the next room, perhaps—or existing only in fantasy, can intervene and instantly sweep away the most serious thoughts, the most important activities, the most lofty aspirations, the most critical responsibilities and demand response *now*. One may wake up in the morning with a long and busy agenda for the day's activities, only to discover that he or she feels an insistent demand for the body of a person of the opposite sex. The day is doomed to be a struggle between the agenda of responsibilities and the paralyzing longing that the sex demand insidiously interjects into every thought and action. The conventions of society and the controls his sense of responsibility exert will probably get him through the day with the agenda discharged in some fashion or other, but he must admit honestly to himself that if he could have suspended or appeased his sexual hunger, he would have done a much better job on the agenda.

Even though the experience I have described in the last paragraph is widespread, many still blind themselves to it and argue that the only real sexual problem is guilt feelings inherited from childhood experiences and inflexible religious norms. Guilt may mess up our sexuality, but even a man totally free from neurotic guilt must admit, if he is honest, that the reduction of guilt feelings does not contribute very much to the taming of the sexual tiger.

Not that the taming of sexuality is an appropriate goal, for a tame sexuality is not a human sexuality—and probably one that is not much fun either. To argue, as I have in these pages, that sexuality is a raw, elemental force is not to say that one should be ashamed of primitive passion, much less try to tame it. The argument, rather, is that the beginning of sexual wisdom is to understand that we are dealing with a power that cannot be tamed. Living with sexuality does not mean eliminating its primal force; it means, rather, understanding how primal the force is and channeling it in directions that are both socially and personally productive.

We are frequently informed that ours is becoming a more "permissive" society in which the atmosphere is much more permeated by sexuality than it has been in the past. Observers dispute whether this is a good thing or a bad thing. The availability of pornographic literature, the use of the naked human form (usually female) as an advertising gimmick, the appearance of "16-mm films from San Francisco" in neighborhood theaters—these are praised by the liberals as a sign that we are becoming more like Sweden and Denmark and damned by conservatives on the ground that we are becoming more like Babylon. (I can't really believe that the liberal defenders of pornography think that the "sex shops" of Copenhagen represent maturity, liberation, or happiness, but to each his own, I guess.) But much of this is nonsense. What makes our world pervasively sexual is not the presence of more or less unclad bodies of the opposite sex, but rather the very presence of bodies of the opposite sex (for that matter, as no one is completely heterosexual, bodies of our own sex too) no matter how covered with clothes they may be. The blatant sexuality of this society, for example, did not arise from the fact that an occasional woman—or indeed, perhaps many women—may appear on the streets braless in a transparent blouse. The real sexuality of the social atmosphere comes from the fact that there are women at all and that they have breasts—no matter how they cover them. However breasts are hidden or displayed is much less important than the fact that the man *knows* that they are there and that therefore this other human being he encounters (even if it is only a transitory meeting on the elevator of his office building) is a potential sexual partner. That is the *real* problem. Any man has powerful sexual hungers, and this woman standing next to him, even for a fleeting moment, is capable of alleviating these hungers, at least temporarily. Of course she, too, has powerful sexual hungers, though she may be less willing to admit them to herself. She, too, realizes that this man next to her on the elevator can provide her with some moments of intense pleasure. The two of them are disciplined, more or less adequately, by social conventions and personal responsibility. He is not likely to rape her, nor is she likely to seduce him, but both know that intercourse between the two of them is a radical biological possibility and one that promises immense delight. The encounter may be brief, the sexual overtones are implicit and perhaps largely unconscious, the latent power is sufficiently well chained that it will not be released; yet, it is there, stirring round the depths of both personalities.

Let us add to this elevator scene elements that are supposed to be part of our uniquely "permissive" modern situation. Let us assume that the elevator is going from the swimming pool to the fifth floor. Let us further assume that the woman is taking the birth-control pill and has no fear of pregnancy. Let us also assume that neither of the two considers himself or herself bound by the old morality "hangups." Finally, let us assume that they are both clad in swimming pool garb, the blatant sexuality of which is somewhat diffused by the openness of the swimming pool environment, but which is greatly enhanced by the close, intimate quarters of the elevator.

These changed circumstances may increase somewhat the possibility of rape and/or seduction—but not very much. They may increase the mutual awareness of sexual electricity between them. By the very fact that the clothes leave so little to the imagination, fantasy may begin to work in a more active and explicit fashion than it might otherwise. In fact, the changed circumstances only modify slightly the fundamental physical and psychological fact of the situation. Both bodies know and both persons know, however subconsciously, that they are alone with someone who could fulfill their sexual hungers. Such an encounter in any society, however permissive or restrictive, is fundamentally the same experience. The surrounding attitudes and customs modify only slightly the primal forces that are at work in such an encounter.

In other words, if we are to live with our sexuality, we must begin by understanding that its problems and its possibilities, its hungers and its satisfactions, are part of the human condition quite independent of particular time and space. There are both problems and opportunities in our own time that are unique, but they only modify and perhaps enhance the elementary human passions that are involved.

Let us illustrate this with another example. A young man sits on the beach, staring dreamily at the water (as young men do when there's nothing better to stare at). A particularly well-proportioned young woman crosses his field of vision clad in the skimpiest of bikinis. Without the young man's having to issue any instructions, his imagination disposes of the bra and the panties, and he enjoys in fantasy the splendors of the girl's unclad body. Behind him sits the puritan. Assuming that he represents the right wing of that movement, we know that he is shocked at what is going on. The girl is a shameless hussy for displaying herself in such a manner! The young man is a dirty-minded punk for thinking what he is thinking! In other times, when people had a sense of decency, such foul things wouldn't occur! (Right-wing puritans always think in exclamations.) If the puritan is left-wing, he will rejoice that in our more progressive day the standards of beachwear are such that young people can enjoy the transient seduction fantasies that were not available to them in the past. (It is worth noting that both the puritan of the right and the puritan of the left are also enjoying the young woman's body, but from the secure perspective of moralizing about the young man.)

But both puritans are kidding themselves. The clock could be rolled back to 1890 and the young woman be covered from neck to toe in the beachwear of that day. It wouldn't matter much. The young man would see her in a socially legitimated form of undress and his imagination would still perform exactly the same operations as would his descendant's in 1970. There would be more clothes for his fantasy to strip away, but the process would be just as quick. In neither case would he be "dirty-minded," though in both cases he might feel guilty about his fantasy. He would simply be a male of the human race who suddenly experiences the presence of a potential sexual partner arrayed in the fashion that indicates availability somewhat more than does ordinary street garb. The impact on him, be it 1890 or 1973, is not unlike being hit over the head with a club.

And in both instances it is safe to presume that the young woman knows that she is in a situation where it is more socially acceptable for her to make her body available for inspection by members of the opposite sex. Both in 1890 and in 1973, she may hesitate about doing this, but she has a powerful need to make men look at and admire her body and so overcomes her hesitation. She, at the same time, has a need to look at and admire the bodies of young men. Whether it be a three-ring bikini or the bathing dress of 1890 is less important than the explicit statement, which we permit on the beach but not on the street, that here is a body that may be available to satisfy my body on the condition that I make my body available to satisfy yours.

As long as there have been young men and women, such encounters have occurred (though not necessarily on the beach), and as long as there will be young men and young women, such encounters will continue to happen. There is a good deal more to falling in love, however, and much, much more to preparing for marriage than such primitive and basic displays of masculinity and femininity. But the powerful if transient mutual desire of the beach encounter represents the radical roots of human sexuality. No matter how sophisticated or how mature or how self-possessed or how casual or how cool we may think our approach to sexuality is, we are all of us basically boys and girls at the beach.

I am not suggesting that these primal sexual

responses dominate every encounter between a man and a woman, or that they are the only important thing in the encounter, or that indeed they need have much in the way of a direct effect on the substantive purpose that has brought them together. Thus, if a man and a woman are working together, there is certainly no biological determination that demands that they sleep with each other or that their sexuality ever need to be discussed explicitly or that there will be any problem in their working together constructively. On the contrary, they may be able to work together more effectively than colleagues of the same sex. I am saying that their sexual hungers are present, their sexual fantasies are at work, their sexual awareness will be active, and they will be kidding themselves if they think that their sexual differences do not have a powerful if subtle influence on the relationship that emerges between them. Their relationship may go far beyond these fantasies and develop in directions that have nothing to do with them; but as members of the human race they must face the fact that such fantasies create part of the fundamental substratum of their relationship, a substratum that may be much more obvious and important in some relationships than in others, but that is never, repeat never, totally absent.

Civilization developed a set of conventions very early in the game that limited the sexual fantasies of most of us to the imagination. Society simply would not survive and hence cannot tolerate a situation in which everyone is free to act on his sexual fantasies. In Norman O. Brown's polymorphously perverse society, not only would nothing ever get done, we probably would end up killing one another. Men and women do not casually rape each other on the streets (and that is the only kind of sex that would really be casual). We have all learned to restrain *that* kind of sexual impulse (or at least most of us have). (The rape statistics—two-fifths of the women in the country have been the victims of attempted rape and one-third have actually been raped—suggest that we are still living in a jungle, indeed a jungle that in this era of "permissiveness" and "feminism" may be more dangerous, rather than less, for women.) That is the only sort of sexual liberation that is complete liberation. Any compromise with it indicates that we do acknowledge in fact that some sorts of convention and restraint have to be imposed on the imperious demands of sexual hunger.

Many societies, and not necessarily primitive ones either, recognize the immense tensions that sexual self-restraint imposes. They compensate for the tension by designating certain times of the year as periods when "anything goes" sexually, when citizens are free if not to act out all their sexual fantasies at least to surrender to many of their normally restrained impulses. The Saturnalia in Rome, the medieval carnival and Mardi Gras (of which the modern ones are pale imitations), and the American New Year's Eve orgy are all times when some of the restraints are temporarily lowered. It is interesting to note, incidentally, that many of these periods of casual sex were, like the beginnings of new years in that new life, born in the midst of a concession to the demanding and sacred power of human fertility.

There are obviously both Christian and humanistic objections to periodic orgies and to the permanent semiorgy of spouse swapping (or "swinging," as it is called in American suburbia). But societies that tolerate and encourage such behavior have discovered an important point; that is, some release is needed for the tensions that build up when sexual fantasies are limited to the imagination. Those value systems that, quite properly in my judgment, object to orgies and to "swinging" must devise alternative measures to achieve the same purpose. Presumably, such measures would have to consist of periodic modifications of the relationship between husband and wife in which some of the tensions that build up due to the normal restraints imposed by fidelity and the ordinary pattern of their relationship one with another can be released. The solution will most likely involve a development of a relationship between a husband and wife in which their respective fantasies can be more adequately expressed with each other at certain times. Obviously, this is an area that must be explored more fully, and it should be with an awareness that the orgy had an important social function for which a Christian and humanist alternative must be found. Minimally, every husband and wife should understand that if they expect fidelity, they must not only tolerate but encourage a sexual relationship in which both their fantasies enjoy considerable freedom to frolic and experiment. Variety seems to be a fundamental part of human sexual hunger. If one does not find it in the marriage bed—or whatever substitutes fantasy may devise—one will be under strong pressure to look for it elsewhere. The pressure is not, of course, irresistible; no one is biologically determined to be unfaithful. However, this book is not concerned with the inevitability of sin but rather with the power of human passion.

To put the matter somewhat differently, a woman who is learning to live with both her own sexuality and her husband's recognizes the fact that he is a sexual being and that every woman, particularly every reasonably attractive woman, is a potential sexual partner. The wife must understand that it is necessary for the health of their marriage for him to believe that, all things considered, no other woman can provide him with more sexual excitement than she can.

Similarly, a man must admit to himself—and it will probably be much harder for him to do so—that his wife must sometimes yearn, in the depths of her fantasies, to have her body powerfully and demandingly caressed by other men. He therefore knows that the health of their marriage requires that his wife realize that, all things considered, no other man can challenge and satisfy her sexually as well as her husband can.

I am not attempting to prescribe tactics to guarantee marital fidelity. My point is that dull sex is not an adequate response to the profound and tempestuous power of sexuality found within men and women, and both husband and wife should understand that.

But even in a genitally satisfying marriage not all sexual energies are drained away. Those who are not married have even more free-floating sexual energy than those who are. Celibate or married, however, some if not all of our sexual energy will be diverted into other channels. Nongenital friendships, aggression, ambition, artistic creativity, altruism, idealism, social commitment are all forms of human behavior that, while they may or may not be sexual in their origins, certainly become sexual in their manifestations because of their capacity to absorb diverted sexual energy. Everybody either sublimates or represses some sexual energy. Living with sexuality involves not merely the diversion of sexual energy but understanding how and why we divert it and exercising sufficient control over the diversion so that the result is not harmful to us or to others. Much of the punishment we impose on ourselves and our friends and families is the result of poorly understood and badly diverted sexual energy. Indeed, even in the sexual relationship itself, energy can be diverted in such a way as to threaten if not destroy the relationship.

Let us examine the problem of the diversion and misdirection of sexual energy in a marriage relationship.

The most obvious thing that can be said about sexual hunger and marriage is that in marriage one has the body of a member of the opposite sex directly and immediately available. There are no legal or moral norms preventing one from taking that body whenever he (or she) is hungry for it—assuming that the other consents (marriage does not confer the right of forcing sex on a spouse without consent). Society condones obtaining satisfaction from this other body, and society tells the other that he (or she) is expected to respond with delight when pleasure is demanded from him (or her).

Furthermore, as time goes on the partners begin to know each other's physiological secrets. A man learns not merely how to arouse a woman but how to arouse *this* woman, or a woman understands not merely what a man's weaknesses are but the weaknesses of *this* man. Also, they have experienced repeatedly the highly pleasurable satisfaction of their hunger through sexual intercourse with each other. Like every other thing a human being enjoys, this satisfaction creates a predisposition for more satisfaction—not merely more generalized satisfaction, but the highly specific, particularized satisfaction that *this* partner can provide. They also realize that assuaging their sexual hunger by making love to their spouse takes a good deal of tension out of other relationships. Direct sexual tension and diverted sexual tension become anger or aggressiveness or bitchiness.

Finally, and most importantly, of course, intercourse is the natural expression of the interpersonal and fully human love that a husband and wife expect to experience with each other and that they both believe is at the core of their marriage. With all of these factors at work it would seem that it would be extremely difficult for a man and wife not to be sexually aroused vis-à-vis each other much of the time. Indeed, one would expect that two such people might even have a hard time keeping their hands off one another, even in public. Everything in their relationship would seem to be straining toward a constant mutual satisfaction of sexual hunger.

But there are other factors at work that not only change the situation but sometimes reverse it completely. First of all, one simply cannot spend all one's time making love. Both husband and wife have other obligations and other responsibilities. They must exercise some sort of restraint if only because other things in life demand their attention and also because a life together in which there was nothing but genitality would eventually become dull. Let us concede that most American couples could probably spend more time on their physical relationship than they actually do. Married sex is too often hurried, episodic, and lacking in elegance and grace. But even if more time could be spent, it is still true that some restraints would have to be imposed. Not all of one's life can be given over to genitality.

Furthermore, there is a need for sexual privacy. One might question whether privacy might have become obsessive in American society, thus generating equally obsessive spurning of all privacy in the communes and in certain sensitivity groups so prevalant in the seventies. It might be much healthier for husband and wife and for their children if there were more room for them to display their passion and affection for one another in other places besides the bedroom. However, intercourse is still a private act, and a desire for privacy may well be a normal aspect of the human condition.

Thus the requirements both of other obligations and of privacy impose even on a husband and wife some limitations of the freedom they enjoy in the satisfaction of sexual hungers. But these limitations— essentially limitations of the external world—are minor compared to those that arise from the fears, anxieties, defense mechanisms, and resentments out of the past and the present that focus on the marriage bed. The need to "get even," the need to punish, the need to protect and defend, the need to keep others at bay all impose immense constraints on married sexuality and divert sexual hunger into self-destructive and punitive paths. I remember an incident that illustrates the pathos of such defensiveness and punitiveness with a special vigor because it has to do explicitly with that symbol of the marriage union, the nuptial bed.

A group of young people I knew were spending several days at a summer resort area. Some of the couples were married; others, a bit younger, were at various stages of courtship and engagement. One night a number of couples were sitting around talking. The only couple in this particular group that was married began to urge their younger friends to think seriously about ordering twin beds when they began to buy furniture for their future homes. For, as the wife pointed out, even though a double bed may look very attractive before marriage, it is a great inconvenience afterwards.

The younger people listened in disbelief. Both the man and his wife were magnificent physical specimens. By all physical and apparent personal dimensions, the couple seemed made for each other. The younger people could not believe that the two of them did not crave the closest possible physical intimacy. Nor could they believe that in their own marriages they could possibly let their spouse have another bed.

In part, what the married couple was saying was merely a statement of sober realism. Sharing a bed with someone else means conceding a considerable amount of convenience and privacy. It is awkward, uncomfortable, and frequently friction producing. It only becomes tolerable when there is a tremendous physical and emotional payoff in such close intimacy. The marriage bed in a way symbolizes the ambiguity of marriage: The sexual passions of husband and wife have absorbed them into a relationship that is both physically and psychologically inconvenient and quite frequently abrasive.

The young married couple, perhaps without realizing it (or perhaps with deliberate intent to punish one another), were saying in effect that in their marriage, the powers of repulsion were currently much stronger than those of attraction. They really couldn't stand to sleep side by side, and the presence of the other's body next to them at night, far from producing delight, was in fact causing disgust.

What precisely had happened is beyond the scope of this book, but the feelings are common enough, even if their expression is less so. In the battle between delight and disgust, our fears, our resentments, our immaturity frequently load the dice in favor of disgust. But our sexual hungers and energies are not thereby eliminated. On the contrary, they are diverted toward reinforcing the hatred and the disgust. Two men or two women who must temporarily share very cramped physical quarters may fall back on old sibling rivalries out of the past to give shape and form to the friction and resentment that build up in their physical environment. But since there is no (or very little) sexual frustration and disappointment in their relationship, only a minor amount of frustrated sexual energy is being diverted into reinforcing their friction. The marriage situation, however, is totally different. Because the whole thing is about sexual pleasure and satisfaction, both husband and wife feel cheated that their expectations are not being met, and resentment opens wide the floodgates through which sexual energy passes to be converted into resentment and disgust, which in its turn leads to even more sexual frustration. A vicious circle has set in that will not necessarily lead either to the divorce court or infidelity but will most certainly result in the extinction of sexual passion. And still the extinction of sexual passion will not lead to the elimination of sexual energy. It merely means that a substantial component of sexual hunger is now going to be devoted to blaming, hurting, and, when possible, punishing the other for what he or she has done. It is not merely that the couple will move into separate beds (and later into separate bedrooms); now they will devote a considerable amount of their lives—and not always unconsciously either—to punishing one another. They no longer have to restrain outbreaks of sexuality; they have to work themselves up to having intercourse at all. What could easily have been an extremely satisfying outlet for sexual hunger has not only failed to be satisfying but has notably increased the frustration and tension in the lives of both spouses.

One cannot readily dispose of a source of sexual satisfaction that has been blighted by resentment and disgust. The body of the other is still there. Part of the personality still longs for it while another part may experience nothing but revulsion at the thought of union. One is trapped, then, in a situation in which there is not only little satisfaction but in which there is ever-increasing dissatisfaction, frustration, disgust, resentment, anger, and hatred. In such a situation infidelity is less a direct outlet for sexual hunger than it is an indirect outlet, which finds its real satisfaction in punishing the other.

One need only look at a marriage in which disgust has triumphed over delight to see how brutal and punitive the sexual drive can be when it is diverted into neurotic channels. Two people whose bodies once ached for each other (and, presumably, still do to some extent) are busily engaged in an attempt to slowly and painfully destroy each other because their longing got sidetracked. They are not only not in possession of their sexuality (few really are), they have let it get completely out of control. In many cases they are not only not capable of passion for one another (save intermittently, perhaps), they are really not capable of passion with anyone, because so much of their libidos has been directed toward hatred, resentment, and disgust.

A marriage in which sexual hunger is displaced by resentment and punitiveness is but the classic example of how we can divert the primal life force of sexuality into self-destructive behaviors. One does not have to go far beyond the two rigid bodies juxtaposed in the disgust-filled marriage bed to find the corrupt businessman or politician getting his kicks out of amassing money; the viciously aggressive lawyer stopping at nothing to win a case, steal a client, or cut down a colleague; the neurotic housewife who turns the children into misfits; or the suburban gossipmonger who delights in destroying another's personality. All these behaviors are clearly a result of the diversion of sexual energy and are at least a probable sign of a frustrated and unhappy marriage.

I do not know what happened to the young people who advised their friends to invest in twin beds. They were in a very difficult and painful time of their marriage. Their relationship could go either way. Disgust or delight could win. They could go on to separate bedrooms and separate lives. But if that is the way they went, God help them—and God forgive them, too. I believe that God did not want them to have separate beds or separate lives, for he made them in such a way that where they really belonged was in passionate embrace with each other just as often as they could possibly find the opportunity, delighting in each other's bodies and being swept along by the primal passion of their mutual hunger. To turn away from the imperious joys of such an embrace denies not so much their marriage vows as the fact of their creation as sexual beings.

Yet even a happy acceptance of one's sexuality leaves a considerable amount of surplus sexual energy unexpended. The advantage of having a healthy genital relationship is that there is much greater likelihood of one's excess sexual energy being devoted to contructive, healthy, creative activities rather than to self-destruction and self-punishment. Those who for one reason or another find themselves in the celibate state must understand that the difference between them and married people is not that they must sublimate while married people do not have to, but simply that the celibate has somewhat more sexual energy to devote to other activities. According to the ancient law of the grass being greener in someone else's yard, the celibate would be inclined to greatly underestimate the amount of sublimation required of the married person. Marriage is obviously something of a response to sexual hunger. Even the most satisfying genital relationship by no means eliminates all the free-floating sexual energy and hunger that possess one. There is plenty of sexual hunger and emotional tension in the lives of a husband and wife despite their fundamentally happy marriage. The celibate who thinks that marriage eliminates sexual hunger simply doesn't know what goes on in the world.

The celibate must come to terms with the fact that he or she is a sexual being. The celibate's fantasy evaluates members of the opposite sex as potential partners every bit as automatically as does everyone else's. He can no more prevent such fantasizing than can anyone else. He attempts to persuade himself that that electric sexual tension in the elevator doesn't exist or that he doesn't yearn to caress the body of the person sitting next to him on the airplane. He is merely kidding himself; worse still, he is engaging in extremely neurotic repression. The celibate may be well advised to impose limitations on his fantasy (and, of course, married people know that they must limit their fantasy lives too—if they are ever going to get anything done). But restraining fantasy does not mean eliminating it, and renouncing genitality for one reason or another does not mean either that one ceases to have sexual hungers or that one is immune from appraising members of the opposite sex as potential genital partners.

The celibate, male or female, has made a decision, hopefully for good and mature reasons, to engage in more diversion of sexual energies than the married person must attempt. In one sense, this makes his sexual posture radically different from that of the married person, but in another sense, restraint, discipline, self-control, and sublimation are part of the human condition and the celibate misses the whole point if he thinks he is the only one who must practice them—or even that it is appreciably easier for a married person than it is for him.

My purpose in this volume is not to defend either the possibility or the desirability of celibacy as an option for certain kinds of committed persons. Obviously, I believe it is both feasible and in some cases admirable; but that is another question perhaps to be discussed in another book. My only point here is that celibates do not cease to be sexual and they have no monopoly on sublimation.

Sexuality, then, whether we be single or married, is a powerful, demanding, barely controllable element in our lives. Wisdom consists not in repressing it, not in dealing with it crudely and casually, but rather in understanding both its elemental force and the simultaneous necessity and frustration in restraining its vigor and drive. At the risk of gross oversimplification, I think one might state the following five rules for living with sexual hunger:

1. We must accept the tremendous power of our sexuality and acknowledge the weakness and inadequacy of our control over that power.
2. We must accept the fact that our sexuality flows

in many strange eddies and currents and can be diverted down dark, hateful, and punitive streams.

3. We must accept the fact that the same ill-controlled and frequently deceptive power that we experience also exists in everyone else.

4. We must accept the fact that casual attitudes, simple formulae, easy answers, and magic techniques are inadequate responses to the fearsome power of sex.

5. We must accept the fact that whatever our sexual posture (married or celibate), hard work and constant effort at focusing energies is necessary both for healthy relationships with members of the other sex and for the diversion of our excess sexual energies into constructive and creative activities.

In a sense, of course, these rules are no rules at all. They are merely a restatement of the problem. But any attempt to deal with the problem of sexual hunger is bound to end up merely as a restatement of the problem. The essence of wisdom about sex is to understand that we are really in trouble when we think we have figured out the answers.

Our unruly sexuality may on many occasions be a burden to us. We might even be tempted to think that life would be much better if there were less passion in it; but, in truth, were we not sexual beings, life would be intolerably dull and inescapably lonely. Guilt over our "animality" is no response to the fact of human sexual hunger—though it certainly has a lengthy historical record for being a popular response. Guilt is an easy substitute for a much more difficult and complicated response—the recognition that our sexuality represents undifferentiated power, the goodness or badness of which depends to a considerable extent on our capacity both to acknowledge its importance and to humbly accept our inadequacies to do anything more than partially contain it.

Is it possible to find in the Christian symbol system anything that will illumine the ambiguity of human sexual hunger? Mircea Eliade, in his book *Mephistopheles and the Androgyne,* devotes a lengthy essay to the *coincidentia oppositorum*. He points out that the myth of the androgyne is widespread in the world's religions as a symbol of man's desire to achieve unity by combining opposites. (Other symbols are the notion of the duality of God, a God of Good and a God of Evil, who in some religions are brothers.) With his characteristic erudition, Eliade finds the adrogyne, or similar symbols, in everything from Goethe's writing to the primitive beliefs of archaic tribes. He summarizes the finding of his chapter in the following paragraphs:

> What is revealed to us by all these myths and symbols, all these rites and mystical techniques, these legends and beliefs that imply more or less clearly the *coincidentia oppositorum*, the reunion of opposites, the totalization of fragments? First of all, man's deep dissatisfaction with his actual situation, with what is called the human condition. Man feels himself torn and separate. He often finds it difficult properly to explain to himself the nature of this separation, for sometimes he feels himself to be cut off from "something" *powerful*, "something" utterly *other* than himself, and at other times from an indefinable, timeless "state," of which he has no precise memory, but which he does however remember in the depths of his being: a primordial state which he enjoyed before Time, before History. This separation has taken the form of a fissure, both in himself and in the World. It was the "fall," not necessarily in the Judaeo-Christian meaning of the term, but a fall

nevertheless since it implies a fatal disaster for the human race and at the same time an ontological change in the structure of the World. From a certain point of view one may say that many beliefs implying the *coincidentia oppositorum* reveal a nostalgia for a lost Paradise, a nostalgia for a paradoxical state in which the contraries exist side by side without conflict and the multiplications form aspects of a mysterious Unity.

Ultimately, it is the wish to recover this lost unity that has caused man to think of the opposites as complementary aspects of a single reality. It is as a result of such existential experiences, caused by the need to transcend the opposites, that the first theological and philosophical speculations were elaborated. Before they became the main philosophical concepts, the One, the Unity, the Totality were desires revealed in myths and beliefs and expressed rites and mystical techniques. On the level of presystematic thought, the mystery of totality embodies man's endeavor to reach a perspective in which the contraries are abolished, the Spirit of Evil reveals itself as a stimulant of Good, and Demons appear as the night aspects of the Gods. The fact that these archaic themes and motifs still survive in folklore and continually arise in the worlds of dream and imagination proves that the mystery of totality forms an integral part of the human drama. It recurs under various aspects and at all levels of cultural life— in mystical philosophy and theology, in the mythologies and folklore of the world, in modern men's dreams and fantasies and in artistic creation (From *Mephistopheles and the Androgyne: Studies in Religious Myth and Symbol* by Mircea Eliade, © in the English translation by Harvill Press, London, and Sheed & Ward, Inc., New York, 1965).

The yearning for sexual union, then, can be seen as but one manifestation of man's drive to break out of the limits his own individuation imposes on him and attempt to achieve a basic unity with the life forces of the universe. Men are impelled toward the woman in the elevator, or toward the luscious secretary, or women toward the man at the cocktail party, or the broad-shouldered male who sits next to her on the bus precisely because union with this other is a means of overcoming separation and of putting the world back together again. This is not just poetry. It is a symbolic description of man's desire to break out of isolation and come into contact with Reality. A sexual partner, actual or potential, is both real and a manifestation of Reality. In a moment of ecstasy, we break out of our fragmented situation and become immersed in the primal life forces of the universe as a fused entity.

Most people don't think this way, of course, and it is perhaps just as well that they don't; but in the sexual union, men and women experience something that might be described on an intellectual level in those terms.

The Christian and Jewish symbol systems, as we noted in the previous chapter, take great delight in using sexual imagery to describe the relationship between God and his people. The very words used to describe the Sinai covenant myth emphasize the intimacy of the relationship: *"I* Yahweh am *your* God"* (Exod. 20:3). They represent the central religious insight of Judaism and Christianity. They proclaim that there exists an "I–Thou" relationship between God and his people. Once that sentence has been spoken all else is commentary and explication. The result of this intimate relationship (and in the Old Testament world, covenants were the most intimate of human relationships), and also to some extent its cause, is a *hesed*, a loving kindness between the closest of friends. Yahweh says that from his people he demands *ahabah*, "love"—but the very same word is used to describe the sexually aroused "love" of the bride and groom in the Song of Songs. Yahweh also proclaims himself *El Kana*, a phrase that we translate badly as "a jealous God" but could be better translated as "a passionate God."

But more than this has to be said. Although little attention has been paid to it, there is some evidence in the book of Genesis to support the notion that the writer of the book considered God to be androgynous. God is not to be thought of as "He," but rather as a "He-She." When a husband and wife, then, seek unity with one another, they are attempting to achieve in their union a perfection that exists permanently in God.

In light of this symbol, then, sexual hunger is not merely a hunger for the Absolute and the Real; it is also a hunger for union between the Male and the Female, which union exists permanently in God. In such a perspective, it becomes possible to say that when a husband and wife who are deeply in love with each other reach the climax of their sexual orgasm, they have achieved something that is, in the strict sense of the word, godlike, because they have temporarily fused the Male and the Female. The *coincidentia oppositorum* has taken place, however briefly, in them, and the primal fracture has been temporarily fused.

Similarly, when our two friends in the elevator feel the brief but powerful electricity that flows from the radical possibility of sexual union between them, they are in fact experiencing a touch of the divine unity. It is not a trace of the divinity that should necessarily be pushed any further, but that they are capable of union with a member of the opposite sex reflects the unity of all things in God. It would seem to me that for the two people the proper reaction is neither to find a bedroom where they can have quick intercourse nor to be deeply chagrined at the power of their own passions; rather, I think, they should be grateful for the spark of the divine that is present in them and the revelation, however briefly, of the power of that spark.

The two of them have other things to do. To spend long hours dwelling on sexual fantasies, to enter a sexual relationship for which neither of them is ready would be inappropriate and foolish; but the brief and powerful experience of their own sexuality is not only not immoral or perverse but a revelation of fantastic (and unruly) forces within them, forces that quite literally can be called godlike.

And the only adequate response to such a brief revelation is gratitude that one has been born a man or born a woman.

A good deal more thought and theological reflection will have to take place before the notion of God as an androgyne will enable us to develop a comprehensive theory that we could call a "theology of sexual hunger." I do not propose to do anything more here than to point out that such a perspective might be far more helpful in trying to explain the meaning of our sexual hungers.

3

Those who take their world view from the Sunday magazines, the national news journals such as *Time* and *Newsweek*, and the television talk shows know that there is a sexual revolution. Unencumbered by much in the way of empirical data, "experts" (and some with Ph.D's) have announced that this is a New Age of Permissiveness made possible by the collapse of the "old morality" and the dissemination of the birth-control pill. Our age, it would seem, is the first one to discover that sex can be fun, and we are all having a rip-roaring good time enjoying it. Most of the "experts" are in strong sympathy with the sexual revolution, though more recently, as the pandemic of venereal disease grips this country, some of them are beginning to have second thoughts.

There are a number of phenomena cited as evidence for the sexual revolution: There is the higher level of promiscuity among college students. Fewer women of the upper middle class are virgins when they marry. There is more "swinging" going on among suburban couples. Homosexuals and lesbians are more aggressive in resisting discrimination and proclaiming that, indeed, their sexual way is the better one. Pornography is more open than ever before and scarcely a serious motion picture can be made without considerable expanses of female anatomy displayed. There is, we are informed, much greater tolerance for sexual deviancy. Finally, some experts see in the communes and in women's liberation the first signs of "the end of the family."

Much of this "evidence" ought not to be taken too seriously. Research into the morality of college students indicates that if there was a change in their sexual behavior, it took place during the 1920s. The only thing that has changed today is their willingness to talk about it. Swingers, communards, and women's liberationists are a tiny minority of the population. The greater tolerance for pornography and deviancy may simply be the current upswing of the unending seesaw of strictness and laxity in man's attempt to impose morality by law. Pornography may be easier to come by now than in the past, but those for whom it was important could get it then if they wanted it. The shapely breasts of starlets in wide-screen technicolor may say more about the difficulties Hollywood has encountered in competing with television than it does about the state of public morality. Nudity in movies merely makes the naked female body somewhat more accessible than it was in the old days of the burlesque houses. (And though the movies lack the third dimension of the burlesque stage, they probably do provide more attractive bodies to look at.)

The Sexual Revolution, then, as it is generally described is little more than a creation of the mass media, much like the Generation Gap, Future Shock, and the Radical Left Student. If one stops to think about it, it is amusing to believe that present-day America is any more permissive than England of the Regency or the Restoration, Paris of the Bourbons, or Rome of the later Empire and the Borgias. Indeed, the information that has recently become available about the sexuality of nineteenth-century England suggests that the principal difference between us and our Victorian predecessors is that we may be more inclined to do openly what they did secretly—and which their predecessors also did openly with far more grace than we, perhaps.

If there be any sexual revolution (among heterosexuals) it is that the birth-control pill makes it possible for more incomplete sexual acts to become complete. The pill also gives women control of their fertility and, together with their employment, freedom to escape from undesirable marriages. The divorce rate has recently tapered off (as my colleague Robert Michaels predicted in 1978 with an econometric model based on the assumptions in the last two sentences) because the rate is now in balance with the number of intolerable marriages in the system.

In fact, the "new permissiveness," the "sexual revolution," the "equality of the sexes," has often meant nothing more than a slightly sanitized version of the *Playboy* Philosophy and has merely provided men with an ideology that makes it easier for them to "score."

There is, however, a real sexual revolution that the media have missed, in part because its complexity does not respond easily to media simplification. Fundamentally, the present sexual revolution results from an attempt to combine friendship with an explicit search for a high level of satisfaction for both sexes in marital genitality—a combination that has been reinforced and emphasized by the Freudian insights about the primal nature of the sexual drive. To put it briefly, the sexual revolution means now that we marry people who are our friends and attempt through mutual orgasm to deepen and enrich the friendship. Compared to this profound change in human behavior, the glimpse of an occasional bit of pubic hair in a Hollywood spectacular is of rather minor importance.

In tribal societies and in ancient cultures, friendship and genitality were rigidly separated. Women and men united to produce children and to maintain the family, but friendship was sought in groups with members of the same sex, in part because of the superstitious fear of something so powerful and demanding as heterosexual intimacy. In the Greek cities, the occasional homosexuality that existed in the friendship groups became commonplace. A man had two kinds of sex life: homosexual with his friends and heterosexual with his wife. The former was a pleasure, a joy, a means of authentic human behavior; the latter was an obligation to family and society. Those men who sought something more in heterosexual relationships turned to prostitutes with whom friendship was possible since such a relationship could be ended easily should it become dangerous.

In the early Christian era, there was a dramatic change in human attitudes. It was believed that in the power of the risen Lord men and women could gain control over their bodies and discipline and dominate their sexual appetites. Sex was no longer an impediment to human freedom because man could be the master of his sexuality. Since there was no

longer "male" and "female" but "all one in Christ
Jesus," friendship between sexes became possible.
But it was friendship without sex. The "coed" monasteries and religious houses of the early church (and
they were viewed with suspicion by such fiery types
as St. Jerome) were attempts to achieve friendship
and community across sexual lines by eliminating
genitality and eroticism from the relationships between sexes.

Some of these agapite monasteries persisted in
Ireland even into the sixth century, and those who
belonged to them argued vigorously against suspicious critics that such joining of the sexes in the
religious life was not only possible but virtuous.
Hereafter follows the tale of the monk Scuthian
(Scothin) and his demonstration of virtue to the
skeptical Brendan (Brenainn). (The Irish writer George
Moore, in his book *The Storyteller's Holiday*, tells
the same story in an uproariously funny contemporary Irish setting. Scuthian becomes a parish priest
and Brendan becomes a chancery office official.)
Vivian Mercier's *The Irish Comic Tradition* (Oxford:
Oxford University Press, 1962, p. 43) gives us this
episode:

> Now two maidens with pointed breasts used to lie
> with him (Scothin) every night, that the battle with
> the Devil might be the greater for him. And it was
> proposed to accuse him on that account. So Brenainn
> came to test him, and Scothin said: "Let the cleric
> lie in my bed tonight," saith he. So when he reached
> the hour of resting the girls came into the house
> wherein was Brenainn, with their lapfuls of glowing
> embers in their chasubles; and the fire burnt them
> not, and they spill [the embers] in front of Brenainn,
> and go into the bed to him. "What is this?" asks

Brenainn. "Thus it is that we do every night," say the
girls. They lie down with Brenainn, and nowise could
he sleep with longing. "That is imperfect, O cleric,"
say the girls; "he who is here every night feels nothing at all. Why goest thou not, O cleric, into the tub
[of cold water] if it be easier for thee? 'Tis often that
the cleric, even Scothin, visits it." "Well," says Brenainn,
"it is wrong for us to make this test, for he is better
than we are." Thereafter they make their union and
their covenant, and they part feliciter.

In the later Middle Ages there emerged in the
Christian countries the idea of romantic love, the
deep, intense, erotic friendship between a man and a
woman without a genital relationship. The great
courtly lovers of the Middle Ages were married, and
apparently they made good enough husbands, wives,
fathers and mothers; but their passionate friendships were not with spouses. The rules of the courtly
love game forbade that these passionate romantic
fantasies should ever end in intercourse. On the
contrary, the whole game was spoiled if the lovers
should ever sleep with one another. The most that
would be permitted, and that only rarely, was fon-
dling, brief nakedness, and a few moments lying
next to each other in bed. According to the rules
of the game, no more was wanted, expected, or
tolerated.

From the modern point of view, both the agapite
monasteries and courtly love were either impossible
or unhealthy. But Herbert Richardson has argued
persuasively that such a judgment may reflect more
on us than on our predecessors. It may indicate that
they understood far more about the complexities and
possibilities of human sexuality than we do. In any
event, according to Richardson, the ideas of friend-

ship without sexuality and eroticism without genitality were necessary preludes to the development of the modern combination of friendship with genitality. As Richardson's title argues, *Nun, Witch, Playmate*—the nun and the witch (the witch being the mirror image of the courtly lover) had to emerge before a wife and a husband could begin to think of each other as playmates. The coeducational monastery and the romantic love of the troubadors were necessary steps in the development of the very modern and very recent idea that marriage, friendship, and the principle of genital satisfaction could all exist in the same relationship.

That, then, is the real sexual revolution of our time. Even in the nineteenth century there was a powerful conviction that marriage and friendship could be combined, but in general, genital satisfaction in marriage was thought to be either unimportant or only accidentally achieved. A woman was thought not to be especially interested in orgasm, and if a man wanted something besides the rather limited genitality that marriage offered him, he was expected first to be thoroughly ashamed of himself and then to guiltily seek satisfaction elsewhere. It is only in recent times—to a great extent after the work of Freud became well known—that we began to believe that it was possible to combine marriage, friendship, and genital fulfillment. Sex became a form of play and mutual orgasm was something that one was to seek principally from one's spouse, who was now not only a friend but also a playmate.

This development is very recent, and while many Americans are willing to endorse it in theory, the practice of spouses as playmates may well be much less frequent. Indeed, it seems a fair guess to assert that the majority of American marriages are more likely to follow the Victorian model than they are the playmate model. Husband and wife are expected to be friends, but both of them are quite reluctant to run the risk of being playmates.

It is obvious that a relationship that combines genitality, playfulness, friendship, and the social obligations of marriage and parenthood is a complex and difficult relationship. Far more is expected of marriage than was ever expected in the past. In our day, it is assumed that marriage will combine the satisfactions that were distributed in several different relationships in years gone by. Men may continue, as they did in Paris of the nineteenth century, to have a wife for begetting children, a friend (usually male) for conversation, and a mistress for satisfactory orgasm; but while society may be tolerant of such a division of labor, the present ideal would still demand that the mistress and the friend and the wife be combined in the same person. Far from eliminating the family, the sexual revolution puts much more emphasis on the marriage union than it ever received in the past. One observer of contemporary sexual mores notes that the modern suburban matron routinely dons lingerie that not long ago only a whore would wear. This is not surprising, because the suburban matron, in addition to her duties as chauffeur, housekeeper, cook, social director, laundress, and mother, is also expected to provide a service for her husband not unlike that which a whore used to provide. Such an expectation introduces into her life a new and challenging and complicated role, one that the social ideal now demands of her, but for which she may very likely be psychologically and culturally unprepared. A whore's lingerie does not a skillful and competent mistress produce. Much less, however, does the recent ideal positing the man as playmate to his wife enable him to bring her the sexual satisfaction to which she now rightly aspires to have every bit as much right as he.

This sexual revolution may make life much more pleasurable, but it certainly makes it more complicated and demanding. The "new permissiveness" is usually casual sex—sex without obligation or responsibilities. In such a union, orgasm is quickly achieved, and the two partners go their ways to "seek new outlets." Such behavior is, for most people, not at all satisfying in the long run, but at least it is easy. It involves no expectations other than quick, uncomplicated fun. The "new permissiveness" in marriage, however, does not so much remove obligations and expectations as it imposes a whole new set of them. The suburban matron quickly learns that while the diaphanous nightgown may be part of her stock-in-trade, it scarcely makes her an effective mistress. And her husband also learns rather soon that simply knowing where to put his hands or his mouth is only the beginning of a sustained erotic relationship with his wife. The combination of sexual hunger and friendship in one relationship may well be an admirable ideal; it is certainly one that is relatively recent. But it is not an ideal easy to achieve or one that most married couples are ready to seriously seek.

There are a number of changes in attitudes— largely as a result of the insights of psychoanalysis— that do facilitate the combination of genitality and friendship. There is probably much more openness in the discussion of sex today than there has been in the recent past, though one is constantly astonished at how many husbands and wives seem incapable of saying anything to each other about their genital relationship. There is certainly more willingness to face explicitly the sexual components of our behavior. There is, I think, more awareness of the mutability of the social conventions by which society attempts to contain the primal sexual hungers of its members. There is certainly more concern about the sexuality of women, perhaps more so than ever before, and it is possible that there is less fear of sexuality than in the past. All of these changes are a sign of progress, although one would be making a mistake to think that they are either as widespread or as profound as some popular discussion would indicate. There are, of course, some people who leap from the speculation of the mass media to practice. They do so generally with little thought and frequently with severe risk to themselves and their partners. But there are infinitely fewer suburban couples who engage in spouse swapping than there are suburban couples who, despite the social emphasis on the new ideal of genitality and friendship and the ongoing public discussion of the "sexual revolution," still find themselves quite incapable of discussing even with each other what happens in bed at night. If the mass media's sexual revolution is not to be taken seriously, the real sexual revolution still has a long way to go before it becomes a pervasive cultural phenomenon. Routine practice tends to trail behind both theoretical ideals and mass-media popularization.

What stance does a modern American take in the face of the sexual revolution? He must first of all acknowledge that the ideal of combining genitality and friendship in marriage is a dominant ideal in his society and that it has a deep impact on both himself and his spouse no matter how far they may be from the ideal in practice. Young men and women approach marriage today with a powerful expectation that they will be able to be friends and playmates. To the extent that this expectation is not met, the marriage is bound to be frustrating no matter how much rationalization may be used to justify the rather low level of adjustment that they achieve.

A woman may have been unconsciously frustrated when she believed that she was not supposed to enjoy sex, but now that she knows she is supposed to enjoy it, the unconscious frustration in the absence of enjoyment becomes quite conscious and explicit, which of course makes the frustration worse. Similarly, a man had no particular reason to feel sexually incompetent if his wife did not have orgasms at a time when the mores ruled out the possibility of full genital satisfaction for a wife. But now that he knows that he is supposed to be a playmate for his wife, his failure to do so is bound to shake his confidence. Thus, there is no escaping the primary responsibility that American middle-class couples have to appraise their own marriage relationship in light of the ideal and ask whether they are moving in the direction of the ideal. There is no point in worrying about the other aspects of the sexual revolution until this primary responsibility is faced.

As for the other aspects of the sexual revolution, the wise man ought to suspend judgment, for as I see it, wisdom means that we neither write off the past nor remain incurably wedded to it. Nor do we take speculative theorizing by self-proclaimed "experts" to be scientific fact.

One of the principal problems of psychoanalysis as a scientific theory is that there is no way to disprove it. It is an inexorable law of scientific argumentation that if there is no way to disprove a theory then there is no way to prove it. If it is not possible to find evidence to refute a hypothesis then it is not possible to find evidence to confirm it. The psychoanalytic spokesman frequently bases his assertions on his own experience with patients, but there is no way one can replicate such experience, and hence no way one can prove or disprove the assertions of the therapist. Indeed, attempts to produce contrary evidence frequently result in the psychoanalytic "expert" asserting that such evidence may be true but collected from people burdened by guilt feelings caused by rigid moral codes created in the past. Or he asserts that the investigator with contrary evidence is himself the victim of his own unconscious drives. Such forms of ad hominem argument may well be effective, but they are not evidence in any sense that the word has in ordinary scientific discourse. The wise man will do well to keep in mind that unless an "expert" states his hypotheses in a way that can be empirically confirmed or refuted, he is offering merely personal opinion—informed, interesting, challenging it may be, but still personal opinion.

There are two implicit assumptions in much of the "expert" commentary on current sexuality. The first is the assumption of "evolutionary enlightenment." It presumes that man becomes wiser and more enlightened with each passing decade and century. Our predecessors were narrow, ignorant, rigid, and uninformed. We are open, enlightened, sophisticated, and informed. Therefore, whatever is occurring today represents not only an intellectual improvement over the past but a moral one too. Breaking away from the old moral tradition is in fact a sign of great human progress. Evolution toward greater enlightenment is not only good but inevitable. The direction of future evolution can be fairly well projected by looking at the young, who are, of course, the most recent manifestation of evolutionary progress. Thus, when relatively small segments of the college population "shack up" in relationships that may be relatively stable, either as a prelude to marriage or as a substitute for it, these young people are eagerly interviewed by magazine writers and their words carefully jotted down as a sign of the most advanced human wisdom.

The second assumption is that of "scientism," which views man as essentially a highly developed animal. The scientism may not be quite so blatant as the serenely arrogant behaviorism of B. F. Skinner, but it assumes that human behavior can best be understood if man is compared with the other higher animals and his actions analyzed independent of the cultural and interpretive schemes that he has developed. Masters and Johnson's research, for example, even though it has unquestionably provided physiological information not previously available, assumes at its starting point that human sexuality can be observed and recorded in the same way one would observe and record the sexuality of any other animal. Researchers like Masters and Johnson would, of course, not deny the importance of the cultural, the social, and the interpersonal as a context for human genitality, but in fact they focus almost entirely on the physiological in their own research, arguing that the physical process of arousal and satisfaction is fundamentally the same between strangers and between spouses whether it occurs in the bedroom or the laboratory with motion picture cameras grinding away in the background.

Wisdom would suggest that both these assumptions ought to be questioned. The wise man is neither an undertaker who wishes to bury completely the traditions of the past nor a miracle worker who wishes to revive them completely; he is rather, as Paul Ricoeur says of the interpreter of religious symbols, a man who is both willing to suspect the past and willing to listen to it. Father John Shea, in his book *What a Modern Catholic Believes about Heaven and Hell*, describes a Christian response to changing cultural values that seems especially appropriate to apply to the alleged sexual revolution:

> There is a strong conserving strain in the Catholic tradition. The Christian is an incurable saver. He drags his whole past with him into the future. He would move quicker if he scrapped many of the things he carried, but he cannot bear to lose an alternative perspective or a possible truth. An ancient religious practice or a dusty doctrine may capture and communicate an undying aspect of the human situation. At the present moment its meaning may be obscure but that does not mean its truth is dead. The Christian hoards wisdom; he is reluctant to part with anything.

The wise man then, Christian or not, is both suspicious of the past and willing to listen to it. He is also suspicious of the present and willing to listen to it. He does not easily give up past traditions, but he is ready to reinterpret them and to refine them when the available evidence seems to indicate that it is time for reinterpretation and refinement. Such an attitude is hard to maintain if, like Alvin Toffler, you believe we are caught in future shock and if, like Margaret Mead, you believe that now we have a culture oriented totally toward the future. Under such circumstances one wishes to jettison the past completely. The position taken by Shea and Paul Ricoeur implies the fundamental unity of human experience and insists that the wise man learns from both the past and the present. Ultimately one must choose either one perspective or the other, and in making the choice one might keep in mind the fact that future believers in the inevitability of evolution toward enlightenment will just as surely and just as categorically reject Mead, Toffler, and all the other "experts" of today as these worthies reject the conventional wisdom of our day. Today's progressive insights become tomorrow's traditional wisdom in the evolutionary perspective. If we expect the future to listen to and respect us, we should listen to and respect our predecessors.

Furthermore, while it may be quite possible to study the sheer physiology of sexual union in the laboratory with only slight attention paid to the interpersonal and cultural context in which the union occurs, the conversion of these laboratory findings into a program for human behavior is not likely to be helpful and may even be counterproductive unless other factors are taken into account. Masters and Johnson make the leap from laboratory to program without bothering to pay much attention to the social, the cultural, the interpersonal, and the value systems in which their "subjects" live. (And their predecessor Dr. Kinsey did this to a much greater extent.)

Scientism and behaviorism find it very difficult to face the fact that man is not just an animal. Alone among all the animals he has the capacity for language, for investing his behavior with meaning and value, for establishing relationships to which his language and the symbol systems it creates give meaning and interpretation that go far beyond mere physical contact. Man's capacity for language and his power of interpretation affect him in two critical ways. It first of all endows him with a capacity for fantasy, which other animals lack, and, secondly, it gives him the possibility, while imposing upon him the necessity, of interpreting his behavior, of assigning it meaning. The refusal of some of the extreme devotees of scientistic philosophy to assign any meaning or value to human genitality is in itself an interpretation. The isolation of the physiological from the other components in human relationships in the Masters and Johnson laboratory is a value decision and interpretation of utmost importance.

It is perhaps understandable that science is fighting the rigid morality of the past, because that rigid morality often stood in the way of the proper development of scientific enterprise. It is also perhaps understandable that science prescind from man as a language-creating, meaning-endowing animal, because his capacity to develop symbols to explain and interpret his behavior for himself and others is extremely complicated and difficult to understand. It is, after all, relatively easy to persuade couples to copulate in the laboratory; in fact, apparently, such an experience can be extremely satisfying on a short-term basis (fantasies about copulating with an attractive stranger in full public view are evidently not rare in the human imagination), but it would be much more difficult to study the complex interaction of friendship and genitality as it takes place in an ongoing relationship where two people are trying to overcome their fears and timidities and grow in trust and pleasure with one another. Of course, until such research is attempted—if it can be done ethically—we only have a limited knowledge of the workings of human genitality. Behaviorists can argue better from a limited knowledge of the sheer physiology of copulation than no knowledge at all. The point is understandable, but the wise man knows that while all things the laboratory researcher says may be true, it still doesn't come close to saying the whole truth.

There is ambiguity and difficulty in standing between the past and the present, being suspicious of the cheap generalizations of both and still listening intently to the insights of both. It is especially difficult to do this when one accepts the serious challenge of trying simultaneously to be a spouse and a playmate, a mistress and a friend. In its most rigid form, the past wisdom says, "All will be well in your marriage if you are faithful to one another." In its most rigid form, some of the modern conventional wisdom says, "If you trade spouses occasionally or sleep around before you marry, or if you become reasonably adept at fellatio, then your genital life will be exciting and satisfying." But neither the simplicism of the mass media nor the simplicism of a narrow behaviorist approach to human activity will deal adequately with the complexity of human sexuality.

The legalism of the past and the simplicism of the present have one important thing in common. They both assume that the problems of sexuality can be solved in terms of whom you sleep with and what particular organs are combined in what ways. As anyone who has pondered his own sexual experience seriously knows, it is not all that easy—and it never will be so long as man has both a fantasy life and the power to interpret and give meaning to his behavior.

4

Being "sexy" is no problem for animals. Most of the time the animal is not particularly interested. When the female is in heat, the male is aroused and their instinctual systems make it quite clear to them how they ought to behave. When the period of arousal is past, "sexy" behavior becomes irrelevant and the instinctual system no longer guides them toward sexual activity.

Humankind is quite different. Its sexual instincts are powerful but not programmed for automatic sexiness. Its fantasy life gives it some broad guidelines as to how to act, but its capacity for interpretation and for definition can impede it and may even suggest that sexiness is somehow or other "dirty."

Humankind, then, has a number of serious problems in coping with its own eroticism:

1. Our sex drive can be aroused at any time. As a result, we have far more sexual energy available to us than do other animals, and we must learn to exercise restraint on our sexual behavior, a restraint that we call "social convention."

2. Humankind's sexuality is set in a matrix of its behavior as a symbol-creating, meaning-giving animal. How we behave depends to a considerable extent on how we define our own sexuality. We are not automatically "sexy": We can only become sexy in a context of meaning and interpretation.

3. Because of our power to create symbols and the permanency of our sexual hunger, humankind has an extraordinarily active, vigorous, and creative fantasy life. Animals do not create poetry, and because they do not they are free from humankind's burden of seeing sexuality everywhere and our profound need for a variety and playfulness in our sexual relationships.

There is little variety in animal sexuality. Some species do have a certain ritual of playfulness that precedes copulation, though it is a ritual that is fundamentally physiological in its purpose and is required to give both animals time to become fully aroused. In the human species, physiological arousal comes rather quickly once the appropriate stimuli are produced. Playfulness in the human sexual relationship, then, is only indirectly physiological in its function and is the result of man's limitless capacity for fantasy, for symbol, and for variety.

If humankind did not have this capacity for variety and playfulness and the need to exercise this capacity, human genitality would be a relatively simple affair. It is evidence of the power of our fantasy life and our capacity to create symbols that something as physiologically powerful as our sex drive can become dull and even monotonous in the absence of variety and playfulness. The attempt to move playfulness out of the whorehouse and into the home and to create variety even in the suburban bedroom is evidence that monotony and boredom are no longer tolerable in marriage. But the challenge that the sexual revolution imposes on husband and wife is a severe one. A routine genital relationship is easy to sustain; one fulfills one's obligations, one gets a certain amount of satisfaction, one does not have to spend time, energy, and imagination maintaining variety and playfulness in the ambiance of one's marriage. One can have sex without having to be sexy.

To be sexy is to create an erotic atmosphere around oneself, to radiate an atmosphere of sexual attractiveness, to invite potential sexual partners, to enjoy playfulness and variety in a genital relationship. The sexy person says in effect, "I am not merely a woman or a man. I am a playmate, a lover with whom you can have all kinds of fun. With me, even some of your wildest fantasies can be enjoyed in reality. I am not just an outlet like everyone else of my sex. I am a challenge and an opportunity."

A second factor, and perhaps a more important one, in becoming sexy is our early childhood experiences. We absorb attitudes toward our bodies and our sex from our parents about the same time that we absorb our language and our fundamental religious beliefs. If our parents are at ease and at peace with their bodies, then we absorb the same attitudes. We are aware of our body's dimensions, its proportions, and its energies. We are confident in its strength and delighted with its potentiality for playfulness and pleasure. We will not be afraid of our body, not very ashamed of it, and capable of using it as a tool of communication with others.

Finally, we become sexy by acquiring the skills

of sexiness. For most, this is a painful and difficult experience. It is not so hard to learn how to act sexy. The Don Juan, the tease, the actor, the model—all are required by their neurosis or their occupation (and quite possibly both) to go through the motions of being sexy. But both the Don Juan and the tease really have no confidence in their bodies and must temporarily build it up by exploiting others. The actor and the model may indeed be radiating an eroticism that they feel in their bones and muscles and to which their intellects and their personalities are committed; but they may also be simply playing a game. Pretending to be sexy is infinitely easier than being sexy. The starlet who so calmly and blatantly displays her charms before the camera may indeed have confidence in her own sexuality and may be eager to enter a love relationship in which she can combine intensity and playfulness—and commitment. But then again she may not, and the body that we see so confidently displayed on the screen may very well contain a personality that is frightened, filled with shame, distrust, and suspicion—capable only rarely of escaping from frigidity. Sexiness is the capacity to communicate our deepest feelings of eroticism to others in a nonthreatening and attractive way. Our capacity for fakery is such that we can seem to communicate with our bodies when in fact we are using them as barriers to keep others away.

To be sexy, then, is to be aware of one's body as an instrument of playfulness and delight, to be able to communicate this awareness to others, and then to commit oneself to a gift of that body in a mutual search for pleasure, delight, variety, and playfulness. Some are fortunate in that either their genetic equipment or their early-childhood experience brings them to adult genitality well equipped to be sexy, but most must learn how; and to learn how to overcome shame and fear, disgust and uncertainties is a slow and difficult process, which cannot be shortcutted by intense weekends of feeling and pawing. Shame is not a demon to be exorcized easily.

Shame is basically a feeling of inadequacy. One is afraid to reveal one's sexual organs because they may not be good enough. Physical shame is intimately connected with human shame; fear to reveal sexual organs results from feelings of human inadequacy. Some feeling of personal and physical inadequacy is probably part of the human condition. Man becomes conscious of himself by individuating himself over against others, and in that act of "alienation," he acquires fears that in his attempts to accomplish union now as an individuated person, he may not have all that it takes. In addition to this "existential" shame, which is part of the human condition, there can be a considerable amount of "psychic" shame. Some cultures and societies greatly reinforce the existential shame by placing strong emphasis on the evil of the human body and the risks of human sexuality. Within these societies certain kinds of early-childhood experience produce intense feelings of guilt and inadequacy. Thus, in contemporary America, despite our happy talk of "permissiveness," many (indeed, most) people approach the physical and psychological stripping that marital intimacy demands with a combination of fear and disgust. Some people manage to overcome these reactions, but others are plagued with them and often use them as means of self-defense for all of their lives. Most of us are not very good at coping either with our own shame or that of our potential partners. This paralyzing shame coexists with an intense desire in our fantasy lives for self-revelation—both psychically and physically. Even if we are able to repress the fantasy of being stripped from our daytime imaginings, we certainly cannot eliminate it from our dreams, and we must admit that while it is a terrifying dream, it is also a delightful one. In the struggle between shame and self-revelation in our fantasy world, self-revelation wins, but in the real world shame is all too frequently the victor.

To complicate matters, there coexists with shame another and fundamentally healthy instinct toward, what I shall call for lack of a better word, "privacy." In most human societies, even those where there is relatively little shame and also relatively few arguments, men and women are concerned about surrounding their most intimate activities with some kind of privacy. This search for privacy, which in many societies is quite unaffected by physical conditions and customs that from our point of view would destroy privacy, may be in part a recognition of the intense power of man's sexual hunger. It also may be a result of the realization that a person's sex is deeply linked to his integrity and his individuality as a human being. The covering of sexual organs would then be merely an assertion of personal dignity and independence.

Privacy, as I have defined it here, and shame need not be connected. They represent two opposing thrusts, one emphasizing human dignity and the other human ugliness; but unfortunately for us the two emotions are tangled together and confused. Privacy is no obstacle to appropriate self-revelation. Indeed, when circumstances arise in which self-revelation becomes desirable, then privacy vanishes; but the motivations that prescribe privacy can be twisted and are twisted by most of us to reinforce shame. A young woman—unless she has that sickness called exhibitionism—is quite properly reluctant to reveal her sex organs to a man with whom she has no desire to share intimacy. She is not ashamed of her sexuality but she does not propose to reveal herself to everyone—a perfectly healthy attitude. But she is plagued by a confusion of privacy and shame. Part of the reason she carefully draws the shade in her room at night is that by so doing she maintains her own dignity and integrity. Simultaneously, she fears the thought of someone's glimpsing her body. To make sure this does not happen, she dresses with all possible speed in the bathroom, perhaps, or even under the covers. It will be hard for such a young woman to adjust to the total change that marriage will work in her life. For with marriage all the reasons for privacy (at least in the narrow sense in which it has been defined here) will be eliminated, yet her shame will persist, and even though she may realize it shouldn't—shame is a powerful emotion that will not be eliminated easily. Shame, rooted in our existential self-disgust, reinforced by our culture and our upbringing, remains a powerful barrier to both physical and psychological self-revelation.

For men in our culture the problem is a bit different. They are somewhat less concerned than women about their bodies being seen by other men (though not completely unconcerned about it either). They are also probably somewhat less disturbed by the physical nakedness that is expected in marriage. However, there is no reason at all to think that there is any less psychic and human shame in men than in women. Indeed, if anything, it may be an even more difficult problem because the active aggressive model provided by our culture for the adult male may make it harder for him to reveal himself than it is for his wife. He may be able to bluff his way through the problem of physical openness a little better than she, but the stone wall of shame is as much a barrier to psychic and human openness for a man as it is for a woman. Perhaps the beginning of growth in love for a couple is the acknowledgment by the man that he is as much troubled by shame as is his woman.

Shame, then, is the enemy of sexiness—shame over our bodies and shame over ourselves. Because of shame some try to get through genital obligations as quickly and as routinely and as seriously as possible. When one is ashamed of oneself and ashamed of what one is doing—no matter how much he or she may be enjoying it—there is little inclination to seek either variety or playfulness; hence, very controlled and restrained attempts to create an atmosphere of eroticism and no wish to communicate the intensity of sexual hunger or the vividness of fantasies, because this would be a form of openness and self-revelation that would obviously repel and disgust others. A man is therefore content to play the role of rough, tough, direct male. A woman is content with being the teasing flirt. Both roles may occasionally look sexy, but in fact there is rather little real eroticism in either of them. A man who does not communicate a capacity for tenderness and sensitivity really isn't very sexy, and a woman who cannot go beyond teasing to clear, direct, and vigorous passion appears erotic only to the most shallow and superficial of potential partners.

Sexiness, then, is a communication of one's nature as a bodily sexed creature. It is erotic self-display. Given the intensity of hunger for sexual satisfaction and the poignancy of desire for love, it is sometimes difficult for most not to engage in erotic self-display. In other words, human beings are sexy creatures, but they can use their capacity for language and meaning to repress this sexiness, to hide it, to cover it, to pretend that it isn't there. Of course, a heavy price must be paid for this pretense; but for many, such a price is preferable to running the risk of ridicule and rejection involved in erotic self-display. It is also easier to solve the problem by denying it rather than by facing the complicated question of when self-display is elegant, tasteful, and effective and when it is repellent, inept, and counterproductive. Both the nudists and the prudes have simple answers to the question, but, as in so many other areas, simplicity is achieved by denying the complexity of the human condition.

One of the most obvious forms of erotic self-display is clothes. In our time, despite the herculean efforts of *Esquire* and, later, *Playboy*, only relatively slight progress has been made toward converting men's fashions into effective means for erotic display. Dramatically colored sports garb and the present, apparently waning, fashion of bright shirts are evidence that men are not unaware that color and variety enhance their sexual attractiveness, but most of the time men do their best to appear as dull, colorless, and unsexy as possible in their daily garb.

For women the matter is quite different. Our society permits them to be much more concerned about varieties of self-display in the clothes they wear. Yet despite the frequently blatant sexual allusions in the garment industry's advertising, much of a woman's concern about clothes is that they be quite devoid of erotic content. Women frequently dress to impress other women with their choice of clothes much more than they do to impress men with their sexual desirability. Thus, clothes, so clearly and obviously a means for communicating both variety and playfulness, are frequently devoid of any explicit erotic intent or content.

The importance of clothes to a woman's own sexual self-image ought not to be underestimated. To put attractive garments on the most intimate parts of one's body is, or at least can be, an act of confidence in the fundamentally attractive and nonshameful nature of these organs. Not only are the clothes attractive; she, as a sexed person, is attractive. Her body is nothing to be ashamed of, but rather something to take delight in. However hasty her glance, she cannot escape the fantasy that what she sees so seductively arrayed in the mirror will be irresistible to a man.

Perhaps it would be a good thing if the woman spent a little more time admiring what she sees in the mirror. The problem for most of us, after all, is rather too much shame instead of too much narcissism. But the image she sees in the mirror is indeed admirable—one of the most attractive sights in physical creation—a sight whose attractiveness she has ingeniously enhanced by her choice of garb. She should admire what she sees. It is very much to be feared that if she is not capable of being struck forcefully by her own attractiveness, she will not be likely to allow others to delight in the scene.

But many women resolutely ignore the possibilities. I remember one disgruntled husband complaining to me some time ago that, for all the elaborateness of her outer garments, his wife's bras and girdles (this was a time when both those garments were considered more mandatory than at present) were tattered and dull. She wore nothing but lusterless and unimaginative white. Her girdles were frazzled and frequently had holes in them, and her bras were held together by safety pins. "She cares a lot about what she looks like to others," he complained, "but she doesn't give a damn about what she looks like to me." It was a blunt complaint and perhaps one that many men would be afraid to speak. The marriage relationship was a troubled one, and the woman's lack of concern about the garments that only she or her husband would see merely indicated the trouble. But she was neither so naive nor so unimaginative as to have any doubt about the message she was sending, and he received it. An aspect of the relationship that could have enhanced its variety and playfulness was in fact doing just the opposite and making it even more routine and dull.

Does it matter to a man what the color of a few ounces of tricot and spandex found beneath his wife's dress is? What difference does it make whether all her bras and panties are white or a mixture of mint, peach, apricot, poppy, coral, etc.? If the only thing that counts in a genital relationship is the coupling of organs, then it doesn't matter; but if variety, playfulness, challenge, stimulation are important aspects of a genital relationship, then the frail garments that stand between a man and the body of his woman are potentially of considerable importance. A woman's use of lingerie to attract, stimulate, and seduce her husband is only an indicator of something much more fundamental and basic in their relationship. If she is not making use of the opportunities the ingeniously designed underwear provides for her, then she should certainly ask herself whether the wasted opportunity is a sign of a much more fundamental problem.

And so, for that matter, should her husband. Our increased knowledge of the sexuality of woman (to be discussed in a later chapter) would suggest that the last garments that stand between a wife's and her husband's body can take on powerful sexual overtones for her as well. The variety of her husband's underclothes can have considerable erotic impact on her. In any event, men's clothing manufacturers have recently introduced a variety of colors and designs into men's underwear that make them obvious garments for erotic display. Multihued tricot briefs are no longer to be found exclusively in the women's section of a department store or in the woman's part of the bedroom dresser. If such colorful masculine underwear continues to be marketed it means that men are buying it in considerable quantity. Thus a catalogue from one very respectable men's clothing firm depicts "ultra print," "rainbow stripe," "criss-cross," and "see-through mesh" bikinis for men as well as a collection of nylon "kaftans," which are described as making those who wear them "sexy" and "irresistible." One is tempted to see a suggestion of homosexuality in some of this, except that the unclad (though modestly protected) women who gaze longingly at the models garbed in the "kaftans" in the same catalogue obviously have something else in mind. Clothes do not the lover make (male or female), and advertising that appeals to the fantasy life may be aimed only at fantasies never realized; but the catalogue indicates beyond all doubt that there is now market value in appealing to the male need for erotic self-display—even if the erotic self is not displayed in very effective fashion to anyone but the self.

It is interesting to speculate that the apparent increase in concern about the erotic attractiveness of the male body may be a result of the increase in demands from women for sexual satisfaction and the inevitable threat to the masculinity of many men that such demands involve. Alas for the complexity of the human condition, a royal blue nylon toga or a rainbow stripe "super bikini" may make a man marginally more attractive to his woman, but it will not make him fundamentally "sexy" or "irresistible" if he has not already come to terms with both his sexuality and hers. Erotic self-display that hides fear, defensiveness, and uncertainty is a poor substitute for real eroticism. However, that men are more aware of the importance of self-display (should one say, "once again"?) is a sign of some progress.

In a good erotic relationship, the two people involved do all they can to make the environment of their relationship conducive to maintaining a high level of eroticism. Intimate apparel, whether a man's or a woman's, can obviously play a reasonably important part in the self-display that creates such an environment. Living with one's sexuality requires both that one recognize the availability of such resources and then use them. But of course the critical question is how to use them. A suburban matron may wear lingerie that years ago only a whore would wear, and her husband may affect garments that only a gigolo would manifest, but it doesn't follow that either partner may be willing to risk a relationship that psychically and physically will take advantage of the erotic potential. The sheer bra and shocking red shorts do not represent much of an improvement over the past if husband and wife are willing to indulge in some forms of erotic self-display in only very restricted and constrained fashion.

From the question of partial undress to that of total undress is only one step logically and psychologically. Nudity is a question of perennial interest and one the complete investigation of which would require a book in itself. Both the nudes and the prudes take extreme positions. The nude sees no problem at all in nakedness, and in his camps solves the problem by denying its existence. The prude, for his part, thinks that under virtually every circumstance a display of the human body is dangerous and evil. The nude sings the praises of naturalness, the prude dashes around with a measuring tape.

Both understand rather little about the paradoxes of nature and of human sexuality—a longing to undress and to appear to others either partially or totally bare, but on the other hand a terrible fear of exposure. (And of course there is a psychological parallel in the revelation of our personhood, in which the paradox of the desire for openness and the desire to hide is even more powerful.) Both opposing urges are strong, both are socially functional, and both correspond to deep personality needs. The solution to the conflict between the two lies not in abolishing one or the other but in determining—with the assistance of social conventions—that under some circumstances it is perfectly appropriate to undress in the presence of others while in other circumstances it is not appropriate at all. The precise nature of the conventions that regulate veiling and unveiling may change and may at given times be either unduly rigid or unduly lax, but the point is that the conventions themselves make it possible to reach agreement on how to combine these two urges.

The bathing beach in modern Western society is a classic example of the functionally legitimated opportunity for dressing and undressing in public. Most people are perfectly willing to display themselves in extremely erotic attire on the beach, while they would not dream of wearing the same clothes to a store only several blocks away. It is not merely that they enjoy exposing most of their bodies to the sun, sea, and sand, though obviously that is part of the reason. The beach is a place where bodies may be seen. A moderately prudish woman who would be very embarrassed if the top button of her dress came open would not hesitate to strip off a terrycloth robe on the beach to reveal a very brief swimsuit. The ensuing delight on the part of those males around her will seemingly not permeate her consciousness. For a brief moment she is engaged in a striptease and she likes it. So do they.

In some societies conventions are far too rigid, and in others they are far too lax. A good deal more relatively harmless erotic self-display on the beach today is far superior to the lack of it there fifty years ago, but whether erotic display on the beach is an indication of how much genital satisfaction is available in a society is certainly open to question. What kind of woman will the girl in the bright bikini be when she is in her husband's arms at night? The young matron who so casually discards her terrycloth robe may find it hard to disrobe with equal casualness in the presence of only her husband. In her stripping at the beach she is in a situation that is not particularly threatening; she can display herself without running much risk to the core of her selfhood. If her eroticism can be as casual in the bedroom with her husband as it is on the beach, then she really isn't pretending. If there are a considerable number of women in the society who can live up to their erotic displays on the beach in their relationships with their husbands, then a pretty convincing case could be made that such eroticism is healthy for the society. But there is some reason to doubt that at the present time such an argument would be valid.

We must face the fact that the nature of prudery in our society is such that for too many married couples inhibitions are so strong that there is probably much less nakedness in their relationship than would be healthy. Despite the powerful and delightful dreams and fantasies, physical self-revelation and self-disclosure are done hastily and almost surreptitiously. Dressing and undressing, activities potentially suffused with eroticism, are about as erotic an experience as eating breakfast. In fact, the variety of dress, semidress, and undress that could occur between lovers is limited only by the creativity of their fantasy lives and time. In practice, for many people whatever nakedness there is takes place only in the bedroom, only fleetingly, and only in semidarkness.

The opposite extreme may be less frequent, but it is equally an escape from wonder and mystery. Casual nudity around the house and in the presence of children is taken by some people to be a sign of progressive and liberal attitudes. It is in fact evidence of the absence of taste and sensibility and perhaps also a subtle seductiveness toward children. People who engage in such behavior make the journey from prudery to exhibitionism without pausing for a moment to consider the possibility of elegance and grace.

But what about nudity beyond the relationship between husband and wife? What about groups of married couples looking for erotic excitement short of swinging in, perhaps, sheltered backyard swimming pools or on deserted sections of beach late at night? What about young people trying to satisfy their curiosity about the opposite sex? What about friends who are not married to each other and do not contemplate marriage, but who feel that partial nakedness or even total nakedness is a form of communication of affection? One must first of all observe that such behavior is not especially new or revolutionary. It has gone on in the past, goes on today, and is likely to go on always. Unlike the nudists or certain kinds of encounter marathons, the "experimenters" described above do not reject social convention; they simply set aside such conventions temporarily and in some privacy. They do so on the grounds that the intimacy of the particular relationship is such that the convention really doesn't apply. As a matter of fact, there is perhaps as much fun in the excitement of violating a convention, in liberating oneself temporarily from official constraints, as there is in the explicitly erotic aspect of such experiences. Nude swimming by moonlight, we are told, can be a hell of a lot of fun. Perhaps it is; indeed, it would be strange if it were not, but there is good reason to believe that such forms of temporary unconventional behavior rapidly lose their payoff in thrill and excitement. It is to be supposed that one must follow one's own taste and sensitivities in such matters. Surely such experiences of nakedness that are not part of a genital relationship are no cure for anything. Nobody's emotional problems are going to be resolved by these experiments. On the contrary, if this kind of behavior is to be both harmless and healthy, it will be so only when fundamental sexual adjustments of the people involved are relatively good—but then perhaps there would be less reason for experimentation. In the present cultural circumstances, nakedness apart from a permanent or quasi-permanent genital relationship would probably not be most people's cup of tea however actively they may fantasize about it. The real problem is not what might happen on the beach in the moonlight but what happens between husband and wife in the privacy of their home. If the young man and woman swim in the nude before they are married, I don't

think I would be terribly troubled by their behavior—
if I were confident that five years after they were
married their psychological relationship would be
such that they were as interested then in erotic
self-display as they were on the moonlit beach. Variety and playfulness between married lovers exist in
the area between psychological openness and trust
on the one hand and intercourse on the other. When
playfulness declines, the other aspects of the relationship may be in serious trouble.

In order to be sexy, to create an ambiance of
eroticism around one's person, it is necessary to
accept the body as good, sexuality as good, our own
personhood as good, and then to understand that
whether one likes it or not one is constantly emitting
sexual messages. The erotic message may be one of
openness, playfulness, and trust or it may be one of
fear, suspicion, and shame; it may be a message of
disgust and revulsion or, finally, a message of weariness and boredom. But there will be a message, and
what it is depends on what is chosen, even though
some refuse to face the fact that they have chosen.

In the final analysis, the question is the capacity
to arouse wonder and create surprise. Weariness,
distractions, problems, home, office, family, school—
all these things bring strong pressure to settle down
to a routine, the ordinary, a life out of which all
excitement, all wonder, all surprise have been taken.
The sexy person is still capable of surprising others
and also himself. In all his relationships there is
wonder, both physical and psychological, because
one cannot ever be sure of exactly what will happen.
Predictability destroys wonder, surprise, variety, and
playfulness.

Let us imagine two lovers. They know at the
beginning of the day that it is very likely they will

make love tonight. Is the routine absolutely predictable, or at the deep end of consciousness are there a
number of questions that delight, amuse, and puzzle
them in the course of the day? The husband, for
example, may be asking, how will she respond? Will
she be hungry and passionate, perhaps even more
aggressive than I? Will she be shy and passive? Will
she want me to take her directly and forcefully—
perhaps even on the living room floor after the children are asleep—or shall I make it a long and involved seduction scene? Will I wait until we get into
bed, or will I begin to undress her in the kitchen?
What will she look like? What will she be wearing?
Will she have on that transparent lingerie in which
she looks so delicious? Will she let me take off her
bra?

And the woman will be semiconsciously dwelling on similar questions. When will he start? Will it
begin even before supper or will he wait? Where will
his hands and his mouth go first? Will he be in one of
those moods when he wants to strip me leisurely?
Shall I turn the tables on him tonight and strip him
first, or will I surprise him with my plan to trap him
at his work in the library when I approach him
wearing only panties and a martini pitcher—or maybe only the martini pitcher? Will I kneel on top of
him, forcing my body down on his?

What is important is not the content of the
questions, for that will vary from couple to couple
and from time to time. The critical point is that
questions like these are still worth asking. If everything that will happen is absolutely predictable and
routine, the wonder and the surprise will have gone
out of the relationship.

It is also necessary that the questions be asked
with a lightness and wit. If the erotic self-display

that goes on between genital lovers is heavy, somber, serious (as it always sounds in the sex manuals), it will also be dull and uninteresting. Playfulness that isn't playful is probably worse than no play at all. Lovers play with each other because it is fun, not because they are applying a lesson they learned in school or proving their masculinity or femininity or doing something that is expected of people of their education and sophistication. The nerves and muscles of the human body, and particularly of the human sex organs, were made to be played with by a member of the opposite sex. While there is obviously no obligation for anyone to engage in such play, it seems utterly foolish for those who are genital lovers not to take the opportunity that is offered them. Yet it is to be feared that prudery, fear, ignorance, and distrust make married love for most people much less playful than it ought to be.

But the fundamental question may not be so much one of sex as it is one of belief. A dull, monotonous, predictable genitality makes sense in a dull, monotonous, predictable universe. If man is caught either by the fates or by chance, if life is without purpose or design, it is a closed and cool universe indeed, and there is nothing to be surprised about and no possibility of surprise; and since there is nothing wonderful going on, there is nothing to wonder about either. Why bother trying to keep wonder and surprise alive amid all the distractions and diversions in one's sexual life when the world is in fact a dull, drab, unsurprising place?

There is, of course, an answer to this out of the Christian symbol system. Father John Shea, in his book *What a Modern Catholic Believes about Heaven and Hell*, concludes by suggesting that we should all approach death with a well-developed capacity for surprise. I think one could push Father Shea's point a bit further and suggest that the essence of the Christian life is developing a capacity for surprise. We really have no choice if we wish to be Christians, because God's intervention in our lives was a total and complete surprise. Yahweh on Sinai caught Israel flat-footed, and the resurrection of Jesus caught the apostles equally flat-footed. Yahweh proclaimed on Sinai and Jesus renewed the proclamation that life is wonderful and filled with surprises, the greatest of which is God's incredible love for us. The Christian can only respond to the surprise of God's intervention by keeping alive his faith in the possibility of surprise and developing his capacity for bringing delightful surprises to others.

It is no poetic exaggeration, then, but strict theological truth to say that the capacity to cause surprise and delight in others by erotic self-display is a continuation of Yahweh's work. It is not merely that by creating wonder in others our faith is manifested in the basic wonderfulness of the universe—the great surprise that Yahweh began on Sinai is continued and expanded.

It is no exaggeration either, then, to say that the wife clad in panties and martini pitcher is imitating Yahweh's behavior. Indeed, if she only has the martini pitcher, she is imitating him even more appropriately, because then both her surprise and her gift are total, just as Yahweh's gift and surprise to us were total.

It will be argued that it would never occur to most women that such revelation of themselves is a model of Yahweh's self-revelation to Israel. It will also be argued that precious few wives will ever work up the courage to create such a surprise.

Both arguments are undoubtedly true, but that is hardly Yahweh's fault.

5

In the previous chapter I suggested that part of the real sexual revolution is the legitimation of sexual pleasure for women and an increase of concern about the social and cultural forces that impede the development in many women of a satisfying genitality. It is worthwhile to summarize some of the research findings that have recently become available. Many people may have reservations about the way the data were obtained, but there seems little reason to doubt their accuracy.

1. It is apparently true that it takes somewhat longer for a woman to arrive at a full state of physiological sexual arousal than a man, but not much longer.
2. Sexual arousal in a woman declines much more rapidly than in the man when the source of stimulation is removed.
3. But in the presence of proper stimulation, a woman can remain aroused and experience orgasmic

satisfaction indefinitely. A healthy woman is physiologically capable of at least two or three orgasms while her husband has one, and under some circumstances she may experience as many as six.

4. The physiology of a woman's genital organism is such that she can experience orgasms indefinitely, with the only limit being physical exhaustion. Researchers report that some women can "enjoy" as many as fifty orgasms in an hour.

5. It is therefore literally true to say that a woman is sexually insatiable. She may be psychologically satisfied with one orgasm but physical satiety in the sense of having obtained sufficient physical release so that there is no possibility of more release apparently does not exist in women.

6. While cultural and psychological variables may make it difficult for a woman to experience either arousal or orgasm, physiologically it is a relatively easy matter to arouse a woman.

These findings run against the overwhelming weight of folk belief, cultural expectation, and the experience of most women. If it is no longer assumed that women don't need or want sex (and I suspect that many men and women are not yet ready to reject that assumption), it is still generally assumed that a woman's sexual needs are less than those of her husband and that she finds it much easier to control her sexual drive. In fact, however, the evidence suggests that a sexually aroused woman "can't help herself" in the sense that her body, once aroused, has both a powerful urge for satisfaction and the capacity for being aroused almost immediately once again. Uninhibited by cultural and psychological barriers, a woman's sexuality appears to be both more intense and more demanding than that of a man.

It is obvious that if a woman's sexuality is so powerful, tremendous cultural and psychological barriers have been built up not merely to contain such driving hunger but even to persuade most women that it does not exist. Such powerful constraints are bound to impede personality growth and cause moderate if not severe psychological harm.

It is not yet clear how restraints on female sexuality came to be, and given the fact that they appear to be very ancient (though there are tribes that do not have them), it may be impossible for us to ever know for certain. Some scholars have suggested that in the evolutionary process the female of the human species ended up with a physiology that left her at all times like the females of other primate species when they are in heat. A woman constantly capable of orgasm and insatiably demanding it would be a tremendous threat to the stability and peace of her tribe—and presumably also to her own health and welfare. As humankind evolved both biologically and culturally and began to organize itself, first into families and then into small agricultural villages, such sexuality became even more of a threat to the fragile structure it was trying to elaborate. It therefore became necessary to develop powerful inhibitions to control female sexuality. The fear of the female, so widespread in primitive tribes, and the powerful taboos imposed on sexuality in this view of things were amply justified by the threat that they presented to mankind's emerging social structure.

The point of view of some militant feminists, that men forced such cultural and psychological restraints on women, is historically and socially far too simple. (It is part of the standard contemporary political strategy of gaining a moral advantage over someone else by saying that as your predecessors oppressed my predecessors so you are victimizing me, and you should do penance by letting me victimize you for a while.) Presumably, men and women both benefited in many respects from a more stable and productive social order. Presumably, men and women both have had to pay a heavy price for the loss of sexual responsiveness in so many women down through the centuries. Presumably, too, an insatiable genitality over which social conventions exerted no control and that suffered no psychological restraints could make life very difficult for a woman.

The explanation is perhaps plausible and interesting, but scarcely documented beyond doubt and probably largely irrelevant to the present situation. The race is not about to return to the forests (there aren't many to return to, anyway). Most women are committed irrevocably to the family and are not going to be persuaded that promiscuity will solve any of their problems. Nor, if the truth be told, are there many women who would think that fifty orgasms an hour is an appropriate goal. Indeed, considerable numbers of them would be satisfied with just one. Whatever explanations we may finally settle on about the origins of the restraints on female genitality, the problem in our day is not to eliminate the restraints completely but rather to facilitate the development of a more healthy and more open attitude toward sex in as many women as possible.

It is clear, then, that a woman's sexuality is a very powerful force when she is aroused. Society and culture have not only imposed necessary restraints on female sexuality but have caused an overreaction to such an extent that many women experience little if any sexual pleasure.

We must be wary about such generalizations. It is altogether possible that many more women have in fact achieved healthy levels of genital satisfaction than are willing to talk about it. The cultural restraints may have applied only to discussion and not to experience. Most of the anthropological literature about Ireland, for example, describes it as a sexually repressed nation, yet one need only read the folktales and poetry translated from Gaelic to realize that there was a very bawdy component to Irish culture.

We are thus entering a period of change when women's sexual hunger and sexual satisfaction are both more acceptable and more expected. For most women this will present a dilemma. Intense sexual pleasure is now all right, but how does one go about experiencing it? In other words, orgasm is now not only the object of legitimate pursuit but also something of an obligation. However enlightened they may be in theory and however convinced by the research evidence that they are capable of sustained and intense sexual delight, women are still caught in the cultural norms of the past as well as their childhood and adolescent experiences. On the one hand, their intellects tell them that they should find out if it is really true that they are insatiable; and, on the other hand, emotional residues of the past warn them that such thoughts are shameful; then the new social application that makes orgasm compulsory demands that they overcome their awkwardness, their diffidence, and their shame instantaneously.

Most women will cope with this problem, if at all, in the marriage relationship. Some "experts" argue that it is debatable whether a context of friendship and love is necessary to develop a satisfactory genital relationship. They point out that the research evidence indicates that almost any man can bring a woman first to sexual arousal and then to repeated orgasm with a television camera grinding away in the background. But then, of course, most people do not make love in the presence of a TV camera, and most people do not have the powerful motivation for sexual success provided by the expectations of the people who are operating the camera. Orgasm, presumably, can take place with almost anyone, but given the fact that human beings endow their relationships with meaning, a satisfactory genital relationship for most of us will require a context of meaning. This context becomes even more important when one (or usually both) partner has a problem overcoming shame, inhibition, disgust, and fear.

But quite apart from the theoretical possibility that a woman can achieve sexual pleasure in other relationships, the truth still remains that most women will experience orgasms in marriage or not at all. Hence the real problem is to improve understanding, insight, and skills—both physical and psychological— in the marriage relationship.

Even though the research of Masters and Johnson and others indicates an astonishing ignorance on the part of many men as to what it takes physiologically to arouse a woman, this part of the problem is relatively simple. If a man is ignorant of what it takes to arouse his wife, it is much to be feared that his ignorance is a matter of choice. Both fantasy and folklore make it perfectly clear what he ought to be doing. He has his hands, his mouth, his penis—what does he think they are for?

The young man on the beach whose fantasy is so eagerly removing the bikini from the girl passing by knows exactly where he wants to put his hands, and deep down in her personality, she knows where she wants his hands to be put and, for that matter, where she would like to put her hands on him. If they should become in due course genital lovers and if he has the courage to follow the inclinations of his fantasy, he will certainly not be very much off the appropriate target. He may need guidance from her as to exactly what he should be doing, but he will certainly know where to begin.

And yet in many cases he will not do so. He may be afraid to experiment; he may be put off by her immediate reaction, a shameful and terrified resistance. Both of them may be trapped in rigid, guilt-ridden morality, which makes them feel that the appropriate actions are "dirty." Perhaps most important of all, the two of them may be afraid to talk honestly and openly about their sexual needs and problems. The relationship goes on, they periodically have intercourse, children are born; but for all the explicit attention they pay to their lovemaking, particularly the question of the wife's satisfaction in the lovemaking, they might just as well not be married.

Conversation between men and women about their genital relationship, and particularly about how the two of them can achieve greater delight and pleasure from that relationship, presumes, at least in most cases, an atmosphere of trust, confidence, openness, and love. A woman can hardly tell a man that he is not doing enough to stimulate her unless she is reasonably confident that their love is strong enough so that the husband will not be permanently offended by such a threat to his masculinity. Nor can a man ask a woman whether he is doing "the right things" to her unless he is reasonably sure that there is enough affection between them for her to overcome her initial reluctance to respond to such frank questioning. There is no doubt that in our time there is less reluctance to talk about such things than there was in the past, although frequently (particularly in the intellectual or would-be intellectual segment of the population) talk in even clinical detail is merely a more subtle form of noncommunication. I am frequently surprised by how many married couples, often after many years of rather unsatisfactory genitality, are able to notably improve both the quality of their sex lives and the whole atmosphere of their marriage after only a few conversations. There is no substitute in marriage for a wife who periodically plays the active and aggressive role in lovemaking, but neither is there any substitute for a man's making absolutely sure that his wife does not feel cheated or exploited—especially since so many women become so skillful at faking satisfaction rather than admit to their husbands that all is not as exciting as it should be.

If even some of the research on feminine sexuality is true (and there is little reason to doubt it), we must conclude that there is a fantastic amount of sexual frustration among American women—some of it no doubt perceived as sexual frustration, much more of it vague and undefined. The frustration is probably even worse for those wives who have read enough to know that they should be enjoying sex, but who are caught in patterns of genitality with their husbands in which they either pretend not to be especially interested in sex or pretend to orgasms they never experience.

A woman has one advantage: Unless she is completely insensitive to her husband's reactions, she knows exactly what it takes to arouse him to the heights of sexual passion. She may never use this knowledge, but she always has it to use if she chooses.

Yet her task is still complicated and difficult. In addition to all her other responsibilities she must engage in a semipermanent seduction of her husband if she is to win the war for his attention from his career. She must overcome his subliminal fears about being an unskilled and inadequate lover—fears that beset many American men. She must teach him the combination of psychological tenderness and physical directness that are absolutely essential if he is to satisfy her. She must bluntly and explicitly guide him to refined knowledge about her physiology. If he is to be an adequate lover, she must make him one—and all the time maintaining an atmosphere that suggests that he is more than adequate, although both of them may know that he is not.

It is not fair that a woman should have to do all of these things. It is not fair that she must assume the responsibility for training her husband to be a lover while letting him think that he is initiating her into the joys of sexuality. But it is much to be feared that in our culture the only alternative for most women is continued sexual frustration.

These facts were made quite clear to me by a couple in their late thirties whom I had known very well. They had married early and produced a brood of children. He was a well-meaning, sincere, and very successful businessman whose knowledge of the physiology and psychology of women was practically nonexistent. He was very sorry about the "emotional problems" his wife had, but he was quite incapable of linking them with sexual frustration, much less with his inadequacies as a lover. Nor, when their marriage began to come apart, could he understand what was going on. When a friend suggested to him that his wife was hungry for attention and affection (and they might have added tenderness and orgasm), he was utterly baffled. He was a good husband and father, he worked hard, paid all the bills, provided clothes, cars, a home, vacations, educations. What more could he do?

I do not think he "played around" with other women, although many men in his situation do. Deciding that fulfillment of sexual fantasies can't happen in marriage, many men (and women) look elsewhere for their "kicks." They feel guilty about their infidelity, but never think that it may be their fault when there are no "kicks" on the marriage bed. In this case, there were many other aspects of the collapse of the marriage, but the genital relationship was both a partial cause of the other problems and a symbol of everything that had gone wrong with their marriage.

After considerable excellent therapy the woman decided that she wanted to save the marriage because of the children and, as she put it, "I still like the goof." In a conversation with me, she described the "long talk" she was going to have with him as a beginning of their reconciliation. I knew them both well and cared deeply about them, so I decided to set aside my sense of delicacy (or perhaps my Irish prudery) to speak bluntly. I observed that a reconciliation meant not a long talk but the renewal of a love affair—or, in their case, the beginning of the love affair that their marriage had only pretended to. "And," I concluded, "love affairs don't begin with long talks."

She agreed that they did not. "What do they begin with?"

"They begin with seduction."

She smiled somewhat ruefully. "I could pick him up at the train station tonight and have him seduced in about thirty seconds."

"Have you ever?"

Of course she had not. She realized it was not the only problem in their marriage, but she also knew enough from her therapy to know that seducing her husband fairly often was an essential prerequisite for saving the marriage—and had been one of the indispensable missing ingredients in their previous relationship.

Only in part was she uncertain about her physical attractiveness as a woman. The major difficulty was that she was unsure how she would be able to cope with the new forces and the new vulnerability in their marriage that seducing her husband in the automobile would introduce—particularly if similar behavior became a frequent part of her life.

It was certainly "unfair" that she was in the position where she had to take all the risk and assume all the burden of beginning to stitch the relationship back together. It was "unfair" that she had to be the first one to put aside the vast amount of residual prudery that remained in their relationship. It was "unfair" that she had to be the first one to make herself radically vulnerable. Perhaps in the future of Western culture this injustice will be done away with. But if this woman wanted a passionate lover for a husband, she had no choice but to accept the unfairness of the situation and drive her car to the railroad station.

She didn't that day. But she did eventually, and as far as I can see, she doesn't seem to regret it.

There are, of course, some—perhaps many—instances in which a woman will need some sort of therapeutic help before she can enjoy sex. In other cases, a man who has not made it his business to discover precisely what it takes to make his wife writhe in uncontrollable joy is not much of a man. He takes his sex when and if he can get it, which is a coward's way out. A man can think of himself as a successful lover only when his wife wants him as badly as he wants her. Indeed, if we are to believe the

recent researchers on female sexuality, the truly successful male lover will have succeeded in arousing
his wife to such a point that she habitually wants
him more than he wants her; and since most men
want their women with barely controllable passion
as often as possible, the thought that they could
want them even more passionately should open up
vistas of endless pleasure and delight. (To quote
Hamlet out of context, " 'Tis a consummation devoutly
to be wished.")

If so few lovers enjoy such pleasure, the reason
may very well be that so few of them want it badly
enough to take the risks involved: those of breaking
away from shame, reticence, timidity, and fear.

6

A recent article in the *New York Times* quoted a number of psychiatrists as reporting an alarming increase in the number of cases of male impotency. The psychiatrists hypothesized that the cause might be the increased demand for sexual fulfillment from "liberated" women. Such demands, the psychiatrists theorized, might frighten even more men who are already troubled by their own feelings of sexual inadequacy. One very obvious way for a man to escape from the insistent sexual demands of a woman who frightens him is to withdraw from the sexual fray altogether by becoming impotent.

In addition, the ideal of "human liberation" pushed by the women's movement can be terribly threatening to a man, not merely because it challenges his already precarious feeling of superiority, but also because he sees his woman seeking for a form of freedom, creativity, and spontaneity that is denied him by the social structure and culture as much as it used to be denied her. If he were any kind of a man at all, he must think, he would be pursuing the same goals of freedom that she is pursuing.

New York is not the rest of the country, and the offices of New York psychiatrists may not be the best sampling points in the nation. The number of cases of psychological impotency may not be increasing. But the New York report merely serves to emphasize something that is well known but rarely discussed—the sexual uncertainties and inadequacies of American males.

The popular myth sees women as more afraid of sex than men are; fear for the wedding-night trauma, shame over physical nakedness, disgust with intercourse, frigidity, slowness to sexual arousal, all these are cited as evidence that women are, to say the least, sexually "slower" than men—despite the data cited in the previous chapter.

Physiological arousal does come more quickly for a man than a woman, not much more quickly perhaps, but somewhat more, and in that "somewhat" there is a considerable difference between man and woman. The average healthy man can get an erection very quickly and experience an orgasm after a very brief period of stimulation—much too brief from the viewpoint of his woman. If all sex was about was erection and orgasm, sexual problems of men would be very few indeed.

But since humankind is a self-conscious, self-reflective, interpreting creature there are other problems for male sexuality, and the very quickness with which man can become aroused can be a serious liability. A man's sexual need and desire is physically obvious. He cannot conceal an erect penis very well nor can he explain it away as the result of cold as a woman can account for hardened nipples. It is clear that a man with an erection has, for the moment at least, most of his physical and psychological resources invested in that erection. The irresistible need to do something about it has taken possession of him. He has lost the dignity, self-control, and restraint that come from being the complete master of his passions. Quite simply, his whole personality wants a vagina and wants it quickly, and there's not much he can do to hide this fact.

But he can be rejected. That which his penis seeks can be denied him, and there is nothing more ludicrous or foolish than a sexually aroused male who is turned down. He has exposed his maleness and it has not been deemed good enough. He has made a fool of himself and there is no way he can conceal the fact.

(Women sometimes report how humiliated they feel when they take the sexual initiative and get no response. As one woman put it, "It is infuriating to go through the whole seduction scene and then be told that he is tired and has a headache and doesn't feel up to it." At least in some cases, there is little reason to doubt that the man is deliberately and not altogether unconsciously trying to show his woman what it is like to experience doubt and uncertainty *every time* you begin a sexual encounter.)

The fear of a failure is an abiding part of the sexuality of many, if not most, American males. There are, of course, a tiny fraction of men who have problems with physiological impotency in their younger years. A considerably larger group have occasional, intermittent, or frequent problems of psychological impotency, mostly rooted in a combination of fear and the need to punish. But many, many more men are harassed at the semiconscious level with a fear of impotency and the related feeling of woeful inadequacy as a lover. What if one finds oneself naked in the presence of a sexually aroused and desirable woman and then is simply unable to get an erection? How utterly contemptuous she will be and how foolish and worthless he will seem. Or what if one does a poor job—a quick erection, a hasty and fleeting experience of intense pleasure, and then the man lies spent while the woman reflects with disgust on how bumbling and incompetent he is as a sexual partner?

Most women, I suspect, are not at all aware of how strong these fears are in their men, and many men permit themselves only dimly to face these fears. Yet, psychiatrists, psychologists, and marriage counselors will insist that such fears are, if not universal, at least pervasive in the society.

In a culture like ours, the position of the male is at best precarious. He is expected really to be two different persons. In the world of career, he is supposed to be vigorous, hard driving, ruthless, ambitious, committed to success ("instrumental" or "agentic," to use the words of psychologists). On the other hand, when he goes into the family psychological environment he is expected to be gentle, compassionate, tender, sympathetic ("expressive" or "communal," to use the opposite psychological terms). He learned these latter skills more or less adequately as a child but always with the realization that when he grew up and became a man he would have to shed them in order that he might begin the struggle for "success." Thus, he was never permitted to be easy in the communal skills as a child, not nearly as easy and relaxed in them as was his sister, and in the years of adolescence and youth he was forced to go through the trauma of acquiring agentic and instrumental skills whether he wanted to or not. Small wonder that he felt guilty about the expressive dimensions of his personality and also feared that they might cripple him in the struggle for success.

In other words, in the world of profession, career, and job, a man is forced to be agentic even though he has little confidence in his abilities in this direction; and in his relationship with his wife and family, he is expected to be communal even though he has little confidence in these skills either. To make matters worse, occupational success is taken in our society to be a proof of masculinity. You prove your virility in one way in the world in which you work and in a quite different way in the marriage bed and at the dinner table. The usual unsatisfactory compromise is something that is not agentic enough for the world of career and not expressive enough for lovemaking. The man approaches his wife like she is a client to whom something must be sold, realizing probably that this is not the way to do it, but not knowing for sure what he should be doing. If you are a virile man, argues the reasoning behind this compromise, a woman will find you irresistible and all you need to do is take her. The net result is a male who in the genital encounter is neither agentic enough nor communal enough. He does not know either when to be strong or when to be weak, or how to take, or how to permit himself to be taken, and you really cannot be virile unless you can combine the expressive with the instrumental. The "stud" may "ball" a woman but that's all he can do. The virile man, on the other hand, knows how to make love, knows how to combine aggressiveness with tenderness, demand with surrender.

No matter how much they may deceive themselves by the locker room version of masculinity, most men know this is the case, and hence feel inadequate when it comes to lovemaking. They will presumably have both an erection and orgasm in the next sexual encounter, but they know that they still very likely will do it "all wrong." There is a difference, the man knows, between a firm, passionate, demanding lover and someone who merely wants to be "laid." A man may pretend that they are the same thing, but deep down he knows better.

The man's virility, then, is put to test in the success world and found inadequate—at least by his own very high standards—because he isn't tough enough, and it is also put to the test in bed, where it is both too tough and not tough enough—and always at the wrong times. How does one read a woman's signals, how does one know when to push ahead, when to brush aside defenses that are not seriously meant, when to tread carefully, when to be gentle, and when to be fierce? A man's reaction is some version of "Damned if I know."

The result for many men is that they take sex when they can get it, when their women dole it out to them. A few moments of passion and tension release followed by semiconscious feelings of frustration and inadequacy. And women, partly as punishment of inadequate lovers and partly for self-defense, become very good at doling out sex in such a way as to guarantee that their men continue to feel inadequate as lovers.

In addition, for all their fierce braggadocio, men are afraid of women, a fear that goes beyond the mere fact that a woman can reject them and can maintain the appearance of sexual coolness and control when they are clearly and defenselessly aroused—though that fear is bad enough. In the very earliest years of life a little boy is warned not to be like a little girl and is under constraint not to associate too closely with little girls lest they capture him and make him like them. Similarly, while he is expected to feel great tenderness for his mother, he is also warned that it is necessary to break away from her "apron strings" in order to become a man. In other words, if you permit yourself to be too closely involved with women and too dependent on them, they may take your masculinity away.

Freudian psychoanalysts refer to this as a castration fear and there can be no doubt that for some men this fear of a loss of masculinity to castrating women is very powerful and very literal. But even where the symbol does not become that explicit, the fear of being "too close" to a woman is still powerful. A man learns early in life that the safest way to deal with a woman is to be self-possessed, a bit aloof, only partially involved. He must keep his options open, certainly psychologically, and perhaps physically, too, and he must also maintain a veneer of mastery, self-confidence, and strength; he may need periodic sexual satisfaction from a woman, and he may also want a wife, but he still must maintain the image to her and to himself and to outside observers that he is not overly involved with her and can be, if he wants, independent of her.

But in fact, his real needs are much different and much more primal for, like all humans, he needs to be both "mothered" and wanted. His wife needs to be "mothered," too, but perhaps not as much as he does, because she learned early in life much better than he did how to both solicit and receive affection, to be covered with sensuous attention, to have every part of one's being, body, and spirit gently and passionately caressed, to experience a relationship that furnishes the psychological equivalent of a hot bath and a warm, dry robe after coming in out of a cold,

damp rainstorm. Mothering is, of course, a powerfully sexual activity, both between actual mother and
child and between adults who provide an ambiance
of psychic warmth for each other. It is not merely
physiological, but the physiological component of
mothering is essential. A child needs to be physically
caressed, and the child in all of us needs periodic
opportunities to assert itself and luxuriate in the
warmth of physical touch. Orgasm may be the conclusion of such a caressing experience (though it
need not), but the caressing experience is important
in itself and not merely as a prelude to orgasm.

One young man I knew complained constantly
that his wife did not "encourage" him enough. She
understood this to mean that she did not exhort him
enough to business and professional success, so she
redoubled efforts in that direction that were already
more than adequate. Nor did he really mean that she
should be available for intercourse. She surely was
ready for that and perhaps more ready than he was.
What he meant, though he didn't know how to say it,
and would have been afraid to if he did, was that he
needed frequent, if not constant, psychological and
physical caressing from his wife. She could not have
mothered him too much—an observation that can be
made about most women in their relationship to
their men. There is no upper limit to the amount of
caressing a man can absorb. The more the better.
And the more direct and physical and sensuous—
and, if you wish, "obscene"—the caressing is, the
better it will be. Does a man need to be "aroused"?
In the physiological sense, generally he does not. He
can have an erection merely at the sight of a woman's beginning to unbutton her dress, and he can
have an orgasm with only the most passive acquies-
cence from her body. But in a psychological sense,

man desperately needs to be aroused. He can be confident enough of his selfhood, his masculinity, his skills as a lover only when the woman has put considerable effort into building his morale, to reassuring him of his work, and encouraging him in his skills. She does not need to caress him in order to have intercourse, but she needs to show him constant affection, to build a psychological atmosphere in which he is self-confident enough to be a lover. He can only be expressive and communal when the strength of her expressiveness makes it difficult, if not impossible, for him to be anything else. The experience of being mothered, then, is absolutely essential for most men in order that they might become confident about their adequacies and strength as men.

And closely related, indeed simply another aspect of "mothering," is a man's need to be wanted. He becomes free to be an imaginative, liberated lover when he perceives that his wife wants him as much as he wants her. It is difficult for many women to convey such a desire to men. Physiologically, their sexual arousal is easier to hide; psychologically, they have been trained to conceal their sexual desires and to keep men at bay by a relative indifference to sex. Their man seems confident enough, though his confidence does not make him particularly satisfactory at responding to her deep needs, but why should she take the risk of admitting to herself and him that she craves sexual union as much as he does?

And yet, the uncertain, hesitant male keeps wondering how good he is, and his confidence in his own sexuality grows as he sees his wife become more and more quickly aroused by him. She does obviously and clearly hunger for him. He really does "turn her on" consistently and not intermittently (and the failure of many women's attempts to become sexually aggressive is that they are not consistent). One can take it as almost axiomatic that a man will not become a skillful lover until it becomes obvious to him that his wife hungers for his body, for, in perceiving that hunger, he perceives, perhaps for the first time, his worth as a male sexual creature.

Being mothered and being wanted can be discussed separately, but in a man's life they are inextricably linked. His wife's affection conveys to him both his goodness and lovability as a male human and also her desire for him. For all their pretense at strength, rationality, vigor, and efficiency, there are few men who do not yearn for the sensual attention of some woman who can simultaneously mother and seduce them. The folk wisdom says that the male must arouse the female, and in a certain physiological sense, this is true. But if arousal means, not merely stimulation of erectile tissues, but also the development of confidence in one's expressive capacities and in the blend of agency and communion in one's personality, then the exact opposite is the case. It is, in most circumstances, the woman who must arouse the man.

At one level of consciousness, most women know that they have been superbly designed to help their husband become more confident of his maleness. Every inch of a woman's body can be a joy to a sexual partner, not merely in intercourse or its immediate prelude, but in the whole ambiance of their lives. In her fantasy life, a woman knows that she can turn her man's existence into a never-ending experience of sensual delight, but in reality she is much more hesitant, in part because of culturally induced shame, but in greater part because of the radical exposure of self, both physically and psychologically, that such an approach to the relationship would involve. What if he rejects her advances? What if he refuses to be caressed? What if he does not want to be wanted, or does not want to be mothered? The point is that on occasion he will, if only because a woman bent on keeping her husband in a semipermanent state of sexual arousal will frighten most men, at least occasionally. What she needs is confidence that she is good enough to break through his rejection.

However good they may be at manipulating a man's fears and insecurities, most women do not even begin to comprehend how fragile their husband's sexual egos are and how deeply they need the most obvious kinds of affection and reassurance. It is a rare woman who can say to herself, "Culture and upbringing have made him more afraid of me and of lovemaking than I am of him. Every sexual encounter between us is more of a risk for him than it is for me." And yet, in most relationships, the beginning of wisdom for a woman is to face and accept these truths.

What can a man do? He cannot talk to other men about his fears of sexual inadequacy. He is afraid to talk to his wife about it for fear she will ridicule him. He may seek out a psychiatrist, though few men do, and he may become impotent to punish his wife, though even fewer men do that. On balance, then, there is little for him to do but suffer through a life of very incomplete and inadequate sex, experiencing orgasm with decreasing satisfaction, and wondering why it seems so trivial much of the time.

Ultimately, there is no escape from such a fate unless a man is able to face his own needs to be mothered and to be wanted, admit them to himself, and then share them with his wife. Such an act of sharing may well be the critical episode in their sexual life. If she ridicules him or is frightened or tries to change the subject or refuses to understand what he is saying, then he surely will never mention it again. If, on the other hand, she is capable of being sensitive, compassionate, understanding, and affectionate, a whole new dimension of their sexual life may begin, for her husband will then realize that she respects him, not less but more, because he can talk about his fears and weaknesses and uncertainties. He will understand, not merely in theory but in warm and passionate reality, that a man who can admit his uncertainties and his fears is not less a man but more a man than the one who cannot. A man who can yield himself to a woman in utter defenselessness is not a weakling or a coward or someone who is asking to be castrated but a strong, confident man who knows that his masculinity will survive no matter what the exposure of weakness and fear may lead to. A woman who does not admire and respect such a man, who does not want to link her body with his as quickly as possible, is a failure as a woman and as a human being. But, of course, one puts the whole relationship in jeopardy by even raising such a question.

How, then, does a man find the strength he needs to plead for tenderness, affection, reassurance, constant caressing; how does he work up the courage to tell his wife that he needs to be wanted; how does he come by the virility that is required to give himself over to the care of a woman in a way analogous to that by which a little boy surrenders to his mother? This question, I would submit, like all the other difficult questions raised in this volume, is fundamentally a religious one because it asks how much one can trust reality, whether the universe is gracious and benign to risk takers or whether the wise and prudent man avoids risk taking, even though the payoff may be great. A man discussing his sexual uncertainties with his wife represents not merely an act of faith in her and in himself but in reality, whether one spells it with a small *r* or a capital *R*. That few men are able to take this risk suggests that there are only few men who are convinced that reality is gracious enough to underwrite such exposure of self. The religious dimension of this exposure of sexual uncertainty may not be explicit, though religious symbols are not very good if an exploration of their meaning does not reveal some insight that strengthens a man's resolve to let his woman see him as he really is.

In the Christian symbol system, the most obvious proof that one does not lose masculinity or strength by exposing one's needs and desires is to be found in Yahweh's making it quite clear how desperately he wants to be loved by his people, and making it clear indeed in explicitly sexual language. If Yahweh can admit that he "needs" the affection of his beloved, then why should any man be afraid to admit the same thing? And if Jesus could weep over Jerusalem because he so desperately wanted the response of that city, would it be a weak man who would weep as he tells his wife how much he needs to be wanted by her? It is hard for a man to concede his vulnerability, to put aside the pose of someone who is always in control of everything, but if God can concede his vulnerability, maybe the admission of vulnerability is a sign of strength and not of weakness.

If most men, troubled, at least in a small part of the back of their minds by their sexual insecurities and uncertainties, do not turn to such obvious religious

symbols for strength, encouragement, and reassurance, the reason certainly in part is that the sexual
implications of the religious symbols have been so
long ignored (despite the fact that sexual imagery is
pervasive in the Scriptures) and in part because
sexual risk taking, underpinned by profound and
clearly thought-out religious convictions, would involve conversion of one's whole style of life. The
ultimate issue, then, is more religious than sexual.
Can we afford to take the risk that reality is good?
Neither the insatiable female nor the uncertain male
is at all certain that such a risk is justified. So their
bed tonight is likely to be passionless or, if there is
any passion, it will be episodic and transient. Technically, perhaps, orgasm has occurred for both of them,
but in that orgasm they perceive, however dimly,
that something much better was possible, but somehow missed.

7

Where do children fit into the sexual intimacy of their parents? The implication behind this question is that children are somehow an obstacle to the playful and passionate lovemaking of their parents; children either as a possibility or as a reality are a potential intrusion into the joys of intimacy.

It is argued that for a woman the fear of pregnancy is always a factor to be considered in lovemaking even if she is using contraceptives. When one wants a child or another child this fear is not important (though the discomfort and dangers of pregnancy are still something that will be on her mind). But if no more children are wanted, then fear of pregnancy is bound to inhibit a woman's spontaneity and joy when she enters a sexual encounter. If in addition she is a Catholic, she may be plagued by such guilt feelings that she cannot enjoy intercourse or indeed anything that seems even remotely related to it.

One must sympathize with those who are caught

in such fear and guilt and one must acknowledge that both feelings are widespread. But about the cause of the fear, at least, nothing can be done. For most women in the fertile years of life, the possibility of pregnancy is always present, however limited the most effective contraceptives may make it. Short of sterilization there will always be a remote possibility of conception. But human existence itself is filled with dangers. It is risky to cross a street, but most people still cross streets. It is dangerous to drive an automobile, but few of us refuse to drive a car. There are some minor elements of risk in air travel, but it is generally acknowledged that fears of such travel are disproportionate to the danger. In other words, if fear of real but minor dangers keeps us from an ordinary human life, we may have a major psychological and religious problem, but that problem is not specifically sexual. If the existential biological fact that one's body is capable of conceiving a child prevents one from enjoying sex, then one surely needs help, but it does not follow that one's fears are natural or healthy or constitute a valid excuse for rejecting all but the minimum possibilities in sexual intimacy.

About the guilt of Catholics using contraceptives little can be said, since this book explicitly and deliberately intends to avoid the current moral debates within Catholicism (in the belief that the issues under debate can only be dealt with when adequate responses to the more fundamental questions raised in this volume are available). The research evidence is overwhelming that most Catholics use contraceptives and have convinced themselves that such use is not immoral. That there may be some residual uneasiness after such decisions is understandable. But if such unease becomes paralyzing even after a careful and conscious moral decision has been made in all good faith, then the problem is psychological, not ethical, and must be treated in the same way as any other psychological problem: When it interferes with normal human life, one needs competent professional help.

I do not intend to defend (or attack) the day-to-day sexual teaching of the Catholic church in the 1940s and the 1950s. That it caused hang-ups in some people cannot be questioned. On the other hand, as a social scientist I must say that most of our general psychological, and specifically sexual, hang-ups come from our family experience, and the church's teachings merely provide convenient reinforcement for problems that had already existed long before we came in contact with the church. The church can be faulted perhaps for not providing the religious vision that would support us in working our way out of our hang-ups. But scapegoating the church is a sign of emotional immaturity precisely because it is an escape from facing the real origins of problems in our family backgrounds.

A much larger question is the problem of the "intrusion" of children. One does not appear in sheer pantyhose and nothing else or begin proximate foreplay in the presence of children. One is not likely to engage in a night of passionate sexuality with a sick child in the house. One must make sure the door to the bedroom is tightly closed before one starts lovemaking—even if one has awakened in the middle of the night. In other words, when there are children in the house privacy means something quite different than it did when there were no children. Like it or not, there are more inhibitions on parental sexuality when children are present. The critical question is whether the man and woman permit these inhibitions to become controlling.

We live in a world of headaches, common colds, sick children, leaky faucets, broken car mufflers, uncertain air-conditioning units, winter snowstorms, late-night telephone calls (to wrong numbers), insanely busy days, pests at the front door, and a thousand other harassments, annoyances, and inconveniences. The question is not whether we can eliminate such distractions from our sexual intimacy or from our whole life experience. The question is rather whether we let them destroy our fundamental life serenity.

There are two ways to cope with the distractions, confusions, and interruptions of our life. The normal way is to respond helplessly to them, to permit ourselves to be buffeted from demand to demand, from distraction to distraction, from annoyance to annoyance. Such a life is one of constant confusion and uncertainty, of wasted motion and mental exhaustion. But it has two distinct advantages: Having given ourselves over to the control of external forces we can argue that we are dispensed from personal responsibility. We can also point to our superior moral worth as evidenced by the exhaustion that results from trying to fulfill our multitudinous responsibilities.

In such a lifestyle children are of course an intrusion on sexual intimacy and so is everything else. Indeed, everything is an intrusion on everything else. It is a life, as James Thurber remarked, of noisy desperation.

The alternative lifestyle requires that one establish a hierarchy of goals and values and arrange one's life in such a way that distractions from high-priority goals are reduced to a minimum. Planning, decisiveness, patience, and persistence are required to live this way—and probably an extraordinary amount of self-confidence and self-control. In such a lifestyle, one is still not completely free from interruptions and distractions; but one has chosen to dominate and control the chaos of existence instead of being dominated by it. Children may still intrude— for it is the nature of children to intrude. But parents organize their lives in such a way that there are times and places of guaranteed privacy and other times and places of minimal likelihood of distraction (even if this means occasional—or even frequent— nights together in a motel).

If one cannot organize one's life in such a way that sexual intimacy is a possibility, the problem is not in fact a sexual one at all but a larger psychological and religious one. If a man and woman say they are simply too busy with children and career to devote much time and attention to sex, they are saying in effect that they have exercised certain options, even though the exercise may have been an implicit one covered up with a disguise of "responsibilities" and "obligations." If one chooses to be disorganized, chaotic, and confused, to be caught in a network of uncontrollable external "demands," then that is the choice one has made. But one then should blame oneself for the absence of anything more than casual sex in one's marital relationship and not the children for "intruding." In that case it is evident that one does not want an expanding sexual intimacy—at least not badly enough to take the decisive control of life that would be essential to make intimacy possible.

I am not suggesting that life can be programmed the way a computer can. The randomness of human events inevitably guarantees that all schedules go awry. A rigidly organized life is the opposite side of the coin of chaos. Both responses to the multiplicity of reality are attempts to avoid the need for mature choice in situations of conflicting demands. Order comes not from detailed schedules but from general guidelines and principles that are applied with ingenuity and flexibility. An organized life means not the absence of confusion but rather the ability to intelligently "play by ear" one's response to confusion—with the other ear listening to a clearly articulated set of values and goals. A lifestyle of control as opposed to a lifestyle of chaos does not mean that one wins all the battles. None of us is that mature, that self-disciplined. It merely means that we win more battles than we lose.

Or to put the matter more concretely: How much long-range planning does it take and how much money does it cost to guarantee a man and a woman a certain number of nights each year alone together with distractions short of disaster most unlikely? How much intelligence does it take to build into a year's schedule of such nights alternative dates in case the primary ones have to be canceled? Is the payoff in their relationship worth the long-range planning and costs? It must be concluded that not all that much planning and not all that much money are involved. If a man and a woman say that they do not have the time or the money or the freedom to take such steps to facilitate the development of their fidelity and intimacy, then they either must claim that life is so harsh and cruel that they have been backed into a corner where sexual intimacy is impossible, or they must admit that they have implicitly exercised options that have placed intimacy low on their list of priorities. One frequent option is to decide in effect that the pain and maturity necessary to exercise control over the chaos of existence is too heavy a price to pay for intimacy—or for any of the other benefits that the assumption of personal responsibility bestows.

The problem then is not the intrusion of children. The problem is rather choosing between responsible control over the circumstances of one's life or abdication of decisive, personal responsibility to the chaos of external demands. You pay your money and you make your choice. And it is a harsh existential reality that even not choosing is a choice.

In the short run, drifting is much easier than choosing. A life of response is easier than a life of responsibility. Blaming the environment is easier than asserting as much rational control as possible over the environment. Lamenting the absence of privacy is easier than taking the rational steps necessary to guarantee some privacy almost all the time and great privacy at least on occasion. Yielding to chaos is easier than imposing order on chaos. Hence it is not surprising that large numbers of people choose the former alternatives. There is great long-run payoff in the latter alternatives but the costs of joining the battle for order and against chaos seem very high—and there is no absolute certainty of victory.

Does the Christian symbol system provide any illumination for the human dilemma of the struggle between order and chaos? The answer is so obvious as to seem almost trivial—except that it is rarely applied to the specific problem of personal responsibility and never to my knowledge to the problem of sexual intimacy.

Primitive man was greatly troubled by the disorder in the physical universe because the forces of chaos threatened his very existence. Storm, drought, disease, marauding enemies could easily sweep in on the tiny, fragile structure of his village or camp and destroy the supports of human existence over which he had labored so long. The social and physical structure of his village barely kept forces of chaos at bay even under the best possible circumstances. He therefore saw the conflict between order and chaos as the primal stuff out of which the world was created and pictured his gods as imposing some order on chaos in the act of creation—although the struggle between the gods and chaos was not definitively won and continues even in the present. Humans cooperated in the struggle on the side of the gods. Plowing the fields, building the village, watching the flocks were acts that shared in the creative activity of the gods because they represented the assertion of order over chaos. They became then necessarily religious acts and the religious rituals that celebrated the existence of the village and the cycle of fertility united man's ordering of his world with the cosmic ordering activity of the gods.

There is obviously a tremendous amount of this ordering cosmology in the book of Genesis. The Hebrews were as much concerned about the battle against chaos as were any of their desert neighbors. But if the setting of the conflict between cosmos and chaos is the same in the book of Genesis as it is in other creation myths, the actors are very different. Yahweh may get upset about the failure of his people to respond to his love, but he does not have much trouble with chaos. Yahweh does not struggle, he dominates. He is not locked in a difficult and almost equal battle; he eliminates chaos with a word. Ultimate victory is not in doubt; it has already been won. Man's work of ordering—represented by Adam's dominion over the garden and his naming of the animals—is not something that is required by the gods to continue the struggle against chaos. It is rather sharing in a victory that has already (in its basic outlines) been won.

One may choose not to believe the revelation contained in the religious symbolism of Genesis: The Ultimate Graciousness of Being has already triumphed over the forces of darkness, chaos, and disorder, and man's ordering activity is a way of sharing a victory. There is still much confusion and disorder—physical, social, and personal—in the cosmos. The revelation (or religious insight if you wish) in the Genesis myth may seem too good to be true. It is not my purpose in this book to argue about the truth of the world view presented in the Genesis symbolism, though I will assert that one can scarcely reject such a world view and make the claim to be Christian. My point is simply that if one believes the underlying religious truth of the Genesis myth, one has very powerful motivation for exercising an option in favor of reasoned and rational personal responsibility over one's life. Chaos can be beaten; it is not necessary to surrender to the forces of confusion and disorder that swirl around us. We can choose, we can take control—at least up to a point. We can make decisions about what is important and what is not important. We can have privacy if it is important to us. Our struggle against the irrationalities and distractions of modern urban life are just as much a part of the ordering efforts of God as was primitive man's building the walls of his village and plowing his fields. The search for appropriate privacy and appropriate times is part of the ongoing battle of cosmos against chaos and we have Yahweh on our side. (The quest for privacy is obviously not the only dimension of the ordering struggle, but it is the one that is particularly the concern of this chapter.)

But is it not still too much to suggest that a man and woman who plan six months ahead of time for a day and a night in the privacy of a motel room in which they can give themselves over to the delights of sexual abandon are participating in God's creating and ordering activity (quite apart from whether any child is conceived during their interlude)? The old piety would dismiss such a notion as a shocking obscenity. The new cynics will dismiss it as religious romanticism. It may well be both. But if responsible personal control over the circumstances of one's existence is necessary for sexual intimacy to flourish, and if the Genesis myth is precisely designed to underwrite the assumption of responsibility as an agent of order against disorder, of cosmos against chaos, then a powerful religious symbol system is available to reenforce the search for privacy, should anyone wish to use the symbols. Religious symbols are options; they impose themselves on no one. If you don't believe the insight contained in the symbol, you don't have to. If you think that the insight is silly, you may say so. If you resent the use of the insight to underwrite the quest for sexual pleasure, that is a matter that is entirely up to you. Only don't say that the symbol is irrelevant to the problems of human life in general and sexual intimacy in particular. The potential for relevance is there if anyone wishes to use it. That the potential has been used but rarely in the past is not the fault of the symbol but of the potential users.

Do not complain to Yahweh, in other words, that the children he has sent you have so interfered with your privacy that satisfactory sex between you and your spouse has become impossible. For he might grow angry and send an angel to tell you to reread the first chapters of the book of Genesis.

The more important question about sexual intimacy and children is exactly the reverse of the one we have discussed in the previous pages: What impact does the sexual relationship of parents have on their children? That the question is asked so infrequently is evidence of how afraid of it most people are. Middle-class parents are willing to make every imaginable sacrifice to provide for the health and education of their children. Nothing is too important to be permitted to stand in the way of a college education. But far more important for a young person than going to college is growing up in a home where sexual intimacy between parents is healthy and growing. However, middle-class parents do their best to avoid facing this truth and try in effect to give their children the impression that physical genitality is something that really doesn't happen between them.

Until very recently the pretense that sex didn't exist between parents was so strong that nothing at all was said about sex, and children learned the "facts of life" everyplace but in the home. More recently some parents (though by no means all or, one suspects, by no means even a majority) have been brave enough to communicate factual information—and if they are "liberal," a wealth of clinical detail—to their children. But few parents are willing to admit even to themselves that the atmosphere of sexuality in the home is immensely more important than "sex education" and usually speaks so loudly that the facts communicated in the frequently awkward "education" sessions are drowned out. Young people learn how to deal with sex by watching how their parents deal with it. The process may not be conscious or explicit (and usually is not), but there are countless cues every day as to what a man is and what a woman is and how they relate to one another. The children couldn't miss such cues even if they wanted to.

Two people who share the same house and the same bed and periodically join their bodies in the genital act (nine times a month on the average in the United States if we are to believe the survey researchers —who know everything) radiate an atmosphere about themselves that is almost palpable. The effects on their bodies and on their spirits of the abrasions and pleasures of their life together are powerful; the tangled network of cues and signs that they are constantly and habitually exchanging make it impossible for them to hide either the general quality of their relationship or the highly specific state of their activity on the marriage bed.

The atmosphere of a marriage is blatant and obvious to anyone who bothers to be sensitive to the cues between husband and wife. Most people train themselves to tune out the signals a marriage emits both because it is acutely embarrassing to witness a frustrating marriage and because if we examine the atmosphere of someone else's intimacy we must face the terribly painful fact that we too are exposing our intimacy for all to see.

Only the perverted would want to have others present when their naked bodies are linked either in warm and deep love or unsatisfactory and transient passion. But the "atmosphere" of a marriage makes clear to the world (or at least to those in the world who can't avoid the evidence) what goes on in the marriage bed, just as though the genital act were taking place in public.

If the powerful and demanding sexual needs of the "insatiable female" are not being satisfied by her man, there is no way she can hide either the fact of his failure or her anger at it. Similarly, if the fears and insecurities of the "uncertain male" are getting worse instead of better, if his wife is making him more afraid of women rather than less, all the bravado and all the beer drinking in the world cannot hide his frustration. It is possible to go through a list of the couples one knows and separate those who clearly have fun in bed from those who clearly don't. Every married couple must realize that their friends can unerringly place them on one side of the list or the other, even if not a single word about sex has ever been said.

If the "atmosphere" of frustration or fulfillment is so clear to friends and even brief acquaintances, how absolutely overpowering it must be to children. If the sexual relationship between man and wife is mutually exciting and satisfying, the children know it, not explicitly or consciously perhaps, but in the depths of their personality. On the other hand, when their parents feel unsatisfied, cheated, and angry over a dull and shabby sexual relationship, the children know it too and this knowledge will have a profound and potentially damaging impact on the children's own sexual development.

Psychiatrists have been telling us this for a long time, but more systematic social science has paid surprisingly little attention to the transmission of sexual role models across generational lines. An exception to this is my colleague William McCready, who calls his field of interest "the transmission of culture." In an ingenious piece of research, McCready has demonstrated the extremely close connection between religious socialization and sexual socialization: A young person learns his world view at the same time and in the same process as he learns his sexual identity. Indeed, McCready and his wife, Nancy, in an article in the January 1973 issue of *Concilium* suggested that it is precisely the rigidity or expansiveness of one's definition of sexual identity that leads one to conclude very early in life that the world is either malign and arbitrary or benign and gracious.

If a child learns that there are certain kinds of behavior that are rigidly required of little girls and rigidly forbidden to little boys, it will be hard for him to believe that he lives in a benign and expansive universe. On the other hand if the child learns (from what his parents do and who they are far more than from what they say) that the fully human person is a mixture of masculine and feminine, aggressive and tender, active and passive, dominant and submissive characteristics, he comes to believe—long before he acquires religious symbols—that he lives in a tolerant and gracious world where there is room for complexity and multiplicity, experimentation and risk taking, openness and trust.

There is an inherent plausibility in the McCreadys' argument and they are now in the process of collecting data that will enable them to nail it down beyond reasonable doubt. Should they do so it will mean that faith and sexual identity are virtually the same thing.

But even before they get the kind of conclusive evidence that good social scientists demand, there can be little doubt that children learn both the fact and the components of their sexual identity and the appropriate style of relationships between the sexes from the atmosphere of the sexual relationship between their parents. What other models do they have to imitate? If being a woman does not mean being like mother, what does it mean? If being a man does not mean being like father, what can it mean? If

playing the role of a husband means something else
than the way father acts toward mother, what could
it possibly be? And if being a wife means a different
style of relationship with a man than the way mother behaves toward father, where is the child to learn
this style?

If a woman deeply longs for the return of her
husband at the end of the day so that he can vigorously
and joyously make her body come alive with passion
and pleasure, both her son and her daughter will
know—without her ever having to say it—that things
are well between mother and father; and even though
the full meaning of what goes on may not be clear to
the children for many years, their mother's confident
need for their father is superb preparation for their
own adult sexual relations.

Similarly if the son and daughter perceive, however dimly, that father frequently caresses mother
and that he often wants to be alone with her, the
impact of the lesson will not be lost on them.

Words, tone of voice, touches, quick smiles, secret laughter, a flash of an eye, a twist of a hip, a
brushing of bodies, a meeting of hands, an occasional pinch or pat or squeal—all of these say far more to
children than does the most clinical and sophisticated "liberal" instruction (not that instruction is out of
place). If a man is sufficiently confident of his role as
a masculine lover that he is able to blend tenderness,
passivity, and gentleness into his personality and
encourage his wife to be sexually aggressive, then he
says things about sex and maleness and femaleness
to his children that they will never forget. If a woman has been reassured of her fundamental lovability
as a woman and if she has been sexually satisfied
by her husband so that she has no doubt about her
own sexuality, if she can mix into her personality

components of vigor, forcefulness, and aggression and can pursue her husband's body with at least as much enthusiasm as that with which he pursues hers, she will teach her children more about sex than they could learn from all the sex education classes and all the marriage manuals in the world (which is not to suggest that classes and manuals do not have their own place).

Most men and women are not prepared to admit to themselves that often they use their children as a shield with which to protect themselves from both the terror and delights of intimacy. There are many different techniques for this particular kind of manipulation. "Obligations" to "the children" are cited as the excuse for permitting themselves little time alone with each other and even for allowing the marriage relationship to deteriorate through lack of care and attention. "The children" are frequently a woman's functional equivalent to a man's occupational responsibilities: Both can easily be cited with self-righteous feelings of virtue for paying little attention and devoting little time to the relationship between husband and wife.

Furthermore "the children" can be a justification for removing from the home environment all traces of eroticism save for those that may occur in the bedroom itself. And even in such connubial privacy weariness allegedly caused by "the children" or the possibility that they might stumble on the scene is used as a pretext for hasty, furtive, and perfunctory lovemaking.

I once encountered what has always seemed to me a classic case of using the children as a protection against intimacy. A couple had undergone simultaneously a severe career crisis and a very difficult period in their personal and sexual relationship. The career crisis had been solved happily and they were going off to a quiet and very remote resort in tropic climes (it was winter) for a week of rest. But, even though their families were willing and even eager to take care of their two children, at the last moment it suddenly became absolutely essential that the children come along. The woman informed me that they had "neglected" the children during the crisis and now they had to "make it up" to them. Her husband was only too happy to agree. What had started out as a "second honeymoon" in which they would have had the freedom and the privacy for sensual experimentation that might have put their sexual relationship back on the tracks was converted— quite literally overnight—into an obligation to "the children" for, as the man called it, "a family vacation."

Of course it never occurred to them that they had a prior obligation to each other and that "the children" would benefit much more from having parents who were physically in love with each other than they would from five tense days under the sun. Or maybe it did occur to them, but they quickly shut such thoughts out of their minds.

And they resented what they had done. For part of both of them desperately wanted the time together for erotic play—and heaven knows they needed it. But they conspired with each other to deprive themselves of such time, blamed each other subliminally for what had happened, and spent most of the trip punishing each other, with the favorite form of punishment being accomplished through "the children." For there is not a parent in the world who does not know how (unconsciously at least) to make children irritable and thus punish his (or her) spouse.

What was unusual about this particular episode was not the technique itself but the fact that it was so ludicrously blatant. The man and woman were terrified of being alone with each other under circumstances where there would have been nothing else to do but make love. They had created a situation in which they would be trapped with each other and then when the chips were down used "the children" as an excuse for copping out. In fantasy they yearned for a "desert island" interlude. In real life, they fled it like it was a contagious disease.

The best sort of atmosphere for children to mature in is one in which their parents are engaged continually in seducing one another. Instead of the question being whether it is fair to the children for parents to devote considerable time and energy to developing their fidelity and intimacy, the question is rather whether it is fair to the children not to. One makes love not because it is good for the children to do so but because it is a source of great delight and pleasure. Yet if one takes or is taken but rarely, there ought to be no doubt that the children will "know," however unconsciously, and that this knowledge cannot help but harm them. (It should be noted in passing that human nature is remarkably resilient. A child can grow up in the most rigid and frigid home and still achieve sufficient sexual maturity to have a happy relationship with a member of the opposite sex—sometimes. But what we are discussing here is not the capacity of the durable human offspring to survive the mistakes of its parents, but the ideal environment for sexual maturation.)

The sexual atmosphere of the home, present and past, is particularly critical when the child experiences the trauma of awakening adolescent sexuality. There comes a night when a girl lies in bed and realizes for the first time (consciously at least) that it is altogether possible that at this very moment her mother and father are engaging in sexual intercourse. If the atmosphere of the family is marked by constant efforts to pretend there is no sexuality in the house and by repressed sexual dissatisfaction and anger, this realization will come as a horrible shock to the girl. The union between the bodies of her parents will seem unspeakably ugly and dirty. If on the other hand the atmosphere of the sexual relationship between her mother and father has always been warm and tender, the girl will still be shocked but the shock will be a pleasant one. She will like her mother and father more not less and—this is critically important for an adolescent—she will like herself more. If her parents have the same feelings she has, then the feelings cannot be wrong and there is no need to worry about them. On the contrary, she can look forward to the day when she can engage in intercourse with her husband, because if her mother does it, it cannot possibly be dirty.

Similarly, the night will come when a young man sees in fantasy for the first time his father making love to his mother. If the atmosphere of his family experience tells him that sex is evil or that it does not really exist or that it is a constant unsatisfying war, he is likely to be violently angry at his mother and his father for being so vile and at himself, both for thinking of the vileness and for not being able to do anything about it. On the other hand, if the sexual electricity between his mother and his father has permeated the home in which he grew up, the boy will be delighted. For if his father can be attracted by his mother's body and if she not merely tolerates but enjoys his attention, then there is nothing evil or unnatural or shameful about his finding the bodies of his female schoolmates a source of constant fascination. And he can look forward with confidence and reasonable patience to the day when he too makes love to one of them.

But there is more to the sexual crisis of adolescence than coming to terms with one's dramatic new bodily feelings. It is essential to know that the feelings are not abnormal or foul. It then becomes necessary to know what to do with them. The adolescent needs an interpretation of his sexuality more than anyone else precisely because he has just discovered it. Sexual rebellion and experimentation among adolescents (and neither phenomenon was invented in 1973) are in fact a covert search for meaning. If a person can't believe what his parents or teachers or church tell him about sexuality, the only way he can find out what it means is by trying it himself (or herself).

Unfortunately young people frequently have good reason for not trusting their elders. For parents (and church and school) have not told them the truth. But worst of all, there has been nothing in the attitudes and behavior of parents toward each other to indicate that they have a coherent system of values that enables them to enjoy the fullness of their sexual passions and energies.

Or to put the matter the other way round, if it is clear that the parents have obtained great enjoyment and satisfaction from their own sexual relationship, the children are perfectly willing and indeed eager to find out what their values are—how they have managed it when so many others have failed. If, on the other hand, it is evident to the children that their parents don't make love all that often, and don't enjoy it that much when they do, there doesn't seem to be any really good reason why they should listen to their parents telling them what is right and what is wrong.

It is as simple as that. All the rules, lectures, warnings, and temper tantrums in the world are no substitute for a mother and father who still obviously enjoy going to their bedroom every night. If mother has frequently come down to breakfast in the morning with a special glow, then her son and daughter will listen to her when she talks about sex and marriage. And if father is still obviously intrigued by the wonders of his wife's body, he will have no trouble getting his children's attention when he begins to pontificate about sex. He may talk like Polonius but his offspring know that he does not live that way and that he can do much better things than talk when he is alone with his wife.

There is great chaos and confusion in the sexual lives of adolescents and young people—maybe no more than in the past, but surely more than enough. One of the main reasons for the chaos is that only a very few young people grow up in the sexual atmosphere described in the previous paragraph. It is another example of the struggle between cosmos and chaos, between order, value, and responsibility on the one hand—disorder, normlessness, and surrender to external pressures on the other. One must order one's own life to enjoy intimacy and fidelity; but having created an atmosphere in one's home that is suffused with a healthy and passionate sexuality, one thereby equips one's children with the attitudes and values that are the raw materials by which they can create cosmos in the midst of the chaos they will experience in their own lives.

One does not love one's mate or lust after the mate's body because it is good for the children—not at least unless one is sicker than even most of the denizens of middle-class society are. A man does not look down his wife's dress and pat her buttock or pinch her thigh when these parts of her anatomy are conveniently present because such actions are good examples for his children. He does these things because they are the obvious thing to do. When they cease to be obvious to him and to his wife, however, the children are going to miss a critically important part of their education.

Nor does a woman keep her body in trim shape, play with her husband's hair, or make the morning and evening kiss a promise and an invitation because such behavior is good for her children. But if she has lost interest in these fundamentals of seduction, her children are being cheated of something that they have a right to: a mother who is not afraid to show that she thinks it's fun to seduce her husband.

8

We live imperfect lives in an imperfect world. Our friendships lack elegance and grace in their self-revelation. Some misread the cues from their lovers. The taking is sometimes too crude and sometimes too timid. The yielding is frequently begrudging and reluctant. The lovemaking is often inept and insensitive. Weariness, nervousness, "headaches," distractions, to say nothing of fear, anxiety, and neurotic regression, all inhibit the generosity of our friendship and the free-flowing of sexual energies. Even the most passionate and skillful of lovers, even the most trusting and confident of friends know that in many of their encounters the balance of satisfaction over frustration is thin, and married lovers often fall off into sleep after their bodies have separated angry at themselves and at each other for what they know was an inexcusably pedestrian performance.

One of the ways in which love grows is by conflict. Such a statement obviously runs against much of the romanticism about love. An "ideal marriage" is one in which the lovers never fight, but beware of the couple that proudly proclaims that they have never quarreled, for either their relationship involves immense amounts of repression or they are archangels.

Lovers must fight. They can only love if they fight; it enhances the quality of their love. Love without conflict is tame, passionless, dull.

In intimacy, powerful forces are released, forces that blend immense psychic and physical intensity. The integration of the genital and psychic needs of two people is an extraordinarily difficult task, because neither individual has anything but limited control over his emotions and hungers. Within intimacy, each must understand and to some extent adjust not only his own hungers and needs but also the hungers and needs of his partner. Love is not the successful accomplishment of a balance among all these surging passionate forces; it is rather the constant effort to strive for a temporary integration of the forces, which will be a prelude to yet more effort. No realistic lovers think that any balance will be permanent, and all passionate lovers know that finding a balance, however transitory, is one of the great joys of their love.

Conflict is an absolutely indispensable mechanism for growth in intimacy. It is the way two lovers disclose to one another the "imperfect fit" in their physical and psychological needs. It is a means for disclosing to each other aspects of their personalities that have previously been hidden. It not merely releases the inevitable tensions that build up in a shared life. It is also a manifestation of love, for conflict between lovers is a means by which they say to one another, in effect, that their love and trust is so great that they are not afraid to reveal to each other their anger and they have no need to hide the raw edges of their personalities.

The most obvious—and the most simple—form of marital conflict is over genitality. Let's say that the husband, for example, is one of those blessed human beings who awaken after six hours' sleep relaxed, refreshed, and instantly ready to face the challenges of the day. Upon awakening he becomes intensely conscious of his wife sleeping quietly and peacefully beside him. She may be a bit bedraggled—as everyone is in the early morning—but in the soft light of morning she seems almost unbearably desirable. He wants her and he wants her now. What better way to begin the day than with a little lovemaking? Sex before breakfast? A fantasy he dreamed of before marriage and one that he can now legitimately fulfill.

What he doesn't know is that his wife, like much of the rest of the human race, is not really capable of human behavior until she has had her third cup of coffee. It is not merely that she objects to sex at 5:00 a.m.; she objects to anything at that hour. She doesn't loathe her husband particularly at that time of the morning—no more than she would loathe the alarm clock, for which she feels a deep and abiding hatred.

Both people knew before they married that not everyone reacts to the early morning in the same way. Both realized that their responses to the alarm clock were different, but neither understood the full implications for their intimacy of this difference. At one point it had seemed very minor; after all, what difference does it make how you feel at five o'clock in the morning? But it turns out to make a great deal of difference, as do all kinds of other small things when they are assembled into a system in which two people brush up against the rough edges of each other's personalities.

Perceive the situation for this young couple. One has to presume they are young, because an older couple would have long since worked out some sort of adjustment. The time before breakfast is for the man the time when he would most like to make love, and for the wife it is the time she would least like to make love or do anything else either. His hungers imperiously demand union, and her early-morning grogginess demands with equal imperiousness that she be left alone. The husband begins to feel that he is being treated like a rapist, and the wife begins to feel used with insensitivity and crudeness.

There are three things that could happen. The husband could accept being repulsed and decide that the early-morning hours are "off limits," that it's too much trouble and not worth the resentment involved. But this does not mean that his desires will go away or that his frustrations will cease. It means that he will resent his wife's prebreakfast frigidity, and this resentment will contribute to a network of resentments that will inevitably exist in any relationship. He will lie there feeling cheated. The filmy nightgown, which should be an invitation, is at this time of the day a mocking barrier.

The woman could give in, as many women do. Yielding to her husband is part of her marital responsibility. If he wants her at such an absurd and idiotic hour, she has no choice but to go along with him; but he is crude and uncivilized, and she makes it quite clear to him that early-morning lovemaking is a responsibility and not a pleasure. She doesn't get anything out of it, and she will give him as little as possible.

Or the couple can fight. In the conflict they will

reveal to each other for the first time what five o'clock in the morning really means to them. The husband will begin to understand what it is like to wake up every morning with a hangover, even if one had nothing to drink the night before. The wife will begin to understand—perhaps with envy—the sanguine serenity of the person who passes from sleep to full consciousness in a fraction of a second. In this exchange of understanding, the two young people will realize that each erred in his interpretation of the other's behavior and learn the real reason for that behavior. What looked like the absence of love or inconsiderateness or insensitivity was really a very simple—though fundamental—biological difference. They are now able to laugh at their differences and work out some kind of balance or compromise. What it will be is something only they can decide, but the important point is that the compromise would have been impossible had it not been for the clarification that emerged from the self-revelation occasioned by conflict.

Not all conflict, of course, ends so happily. (And this one may not either. Those biological differences will persist and compromises will have to be made and remade.) One can take it as axiomatic that the longer the conflict is put off, the more likely it is that the pain, anger, and resentment will blind lovers to the self-revelation in a conflict situation. Their fight will not be an attempt to communicate and understand, to clarify and resolve, so much as an attempt to hurt and punish. The critical point in the conflict, of course, is the laughter, for laughter is a turning point when passionate anger is transformed into passionate love. Laughter occurs at the moment when self-revelation is effectively communicated. The two lovers say in effect, "Oh, that's what you mean!" And however violent the fight may have been, effective self-revelation reveals that the issue is relatively minor. Any difference is relatively minor when compared to the fear that love no longer exists. The conflict ritual permits the two lovers to assert their fear that there is no love, to discover that the cause of tension is much less important, laugh at its relative triviality, and then take steps to eliminate it if possible or at least to integrate it into their lives.

The wife in our parable will never be as wide awake as her husband in the early morning, and he will never be as groggy as she at that time; but they can come to understand each other's responses and to realize that they do not call into question their basic love for each other. They will both have to adjust; they will both have to modify their behavior; they will both have to act against powerful physical feelings on occasion. But neither will demand of the other that they stop being what they are.

The husband will decide that early-morning sex, however delightful, is something that will not occur as frequently as he would like. It will happen sometimes, but, all things considered, it would be better for him to seek other times for prime sexual activity.

The wife, on the other hand, will comprehend that for a man whose physiology is like that of her husband, love before breakfast is important and meaningful. At least some of the time, his desire for early-morning sex is reasonable. She knows now that, having understood their different responses to the alarm clock, he will want to make love at that hour only when his sexual hungers are extremely strong, and when he feels that way about her, she will be not only willing to respond but eager to do so even if the world and her head are both dull, leaden masses. More than that, since she is a smart woman, she will occasionally pick a morning and set out to seduce her husband when he least expects it. She knows that if he goes to work with an experience like that fresh in his mind, he will be only too eager to get home in the evening. A time of such obvious sexual vulnerability in her husband is simply too good an opportunity for a wife who is both clever and loving to pass up.

The example is both comic and elementary. Comic because the mismatch of the physiology of sleeping and waking in the couple is ludicrous. It is one of God's little jokes that at first is not very funny, but once they have faced it and resolved it, it becomes as hilarious to them as it apparently is to God. It is elementary because the differences between the man and woman are simply physiological; they are not (at least necessarily) connected with personality differences rooted in their childhood experiences. The conflict is not an easy one to solve. No conflict in intimacy is easy to solve, but it is much easier to resolve than other, more complicated ones. The pattern of possible solutions is always the same. Either the husband or the wife gives in or they have a fight in which they reveal the reasons for the tension and move toward resolution.

What is important in the marriage is that the couple develop a style and a ritual in which conflict can be waged as often as is necessary without threatening the structure of the marriage. However difficult it may be to develop ritualized ways of dealing with conflict, such rituals are still necessary. A classic example of ritualized conflict in American society is the collective bargaining situation. Management and labor need each other in the economic sphere as much as the husband and wife do in the domestic sphere. Tensions build up between them in the course of a contract. The renegotiation period is a time of tension release, of angry threats, loud warnings, harsh and bitter words. Despite the rhetoric and an occasional well-publicized strike, most contracts are renegotiated successfully and management and labor settle down to another several years of peaceful cooperation. The rituals are not unimportant. They provide for a release of anger, they clarify the situation, they make needs and problems explicit; but both sides know that the fundamental relationship between the union and the company is much too important for both of them to call it into ultimate question. Even if there is a strike, both sides know that it will be settled.

A ritual for conflict, then, must be developed in any relationship. The ritual does not mean that the conflict is not real; it means that the two partners have evolved a mechanism for dealing with tension that allows them to simultaneously express their anger and indicate to each other that the fundamental relationship is not in jeopardy. The style depends on the people involved. The ritual for some people seems to involve constant bickering, which in other couples would surely indicate that the marriage was in deep trouble, but for them it is a means of communicating with each other that reinforces the marriage union rather than threatens it. In other families conflict ritual involves much shouting and violent language. (I have been led to believe by some of my colleagues that in Jewish families this is the most appropriate and desirable—and enjoyable—form of family conflict.) In other relationships the rhetoric of conflict and conflict resolution is much milder. On the whole it seems to me (and here I may be betraying my Irish familial background) that peace is better than shouting, but shouting is infinitely better than silence, and at times may be absolutely essential.

Conflict in intimate relationships ought not to be limited to pyrotechnic interludes. It should be an ongoing part of the relationship. Lovers must confront each other constantly in the process of self-revelation and self-disclosure. Most of the time, confrontation goes on at a low key. The ritual of conflict in the relationship has been so arranged that minor problems and tensions can be handled almost automatically and implicitly. When a problem is minor and when it is major, when it can be solved in the routine of day-to-day confrontation and when it requires a slam-bang mammoth confrontation, depends upon the people involved and their progress in emitting and receiving recognizable cues. Like everything else in intimacy, skill in resolving conflict is only incompletely learned and only imperfectly exercised. Like every other skill, the lovers must always strive to improve their skills at conflict.

In some of the oversimplified versions of group dynamics theory that are currently being practiced, the word *confrontation* has come to mean brutal, vicious, thoughtless attacks on other people. The confrontations so applauded by the sensitivity cults are absolutely disastrous for any relationship, especially for an intimate one. There must be skill and tact and tenderness in every confrontation between lovers.

But it does not follow that in confrontation one pulls punches. If confrontation is to be tactful and tender, it also must be direct, sincere, and to the point. Sometimes I think the appeal of the overkill of the sensitivity cults is that it provides an escape from the much more complicated task of combining directness and tenderness in the confrontation situation.

A confrontation is a demand for the best in the other. It says in effect, "I chose you for a spouse (or a friend) because I saw in you certain admirable qualities. I will not settle for anything less than those qualities. You are a person who is capable of excellence, and it is excellence that I want and nothing else."

The need for confrontation is most obvious in the genital relationship. I knew once of a woman—obviously and clearly frustrated in the early years of her marriage—who presented her husband with a book on sexual techniques as a hint that he had quite a bit to learn about how to sexually satisfy her. He resolutely refused to look at it. Obviously, she should have been much more direct and blunt. She should have told him in no uncertain terms that she needed much more from him. She had chosen him as a husband, after all, because she believed that he had the strong masculine capacity to bring her to the fullness of sexual pleasure. He was not doing this. He was cheating her—however unintentionally—probably because he was afraid to experiment, afraid to risk himself in sex play that he feared she might reject. He needed to be encouraged to become much more demanding and challenging on the marriage bed, but he would not be so encouraged unless it was clear that not only did she want him to do so but that she absolutely demanded that he begin to enjoy her body and to bring enjoyment to it in a far more elaborate way than he had done thus far. I fear that merely giving him a book to read was something less than the vigorous confrontation that the two of them needed.

In another and exactly opposite situation, a husband had married a woman who was certainly not frigid but she "didn't get much out of sex." As her husband complained, "She always closes her eyes when we are making love." It was time for him to make it perfectly clear to her that he married her, at least in part, because he wanted her body—all of it, not just the minor part of it that was offered to him in their unsatisfactory lovemaking. He would simply not tolerate her foolish anxieties and scruples. I am afraid, however, that his tactics were just the opposite. If she wasn't getting much out of sex, then it didn't seem appropriate that he should get much out of it either, and so the two of them sought satisfaction in other aspects of their relationship and pretended that what went on in bed at night was not all that important.

Both these stories are so typical as to be normal. Sexual adjustment in both couples was poor because there was no effective communication about sexual needs, desires, problems, and fears. In neither case did the husband have any clear confidence in his ability to arouse his wife and hence hadn't even really tried. In both cases, the wife who desperately wanted to be aroused was incapable of bluntly telling her husband that his techniques in lovemaking were not up to his obvious masculine strengths. As a result, there was no satisfaction, no confrontation, no resolution, and, increasingly, no sex.

Confrontation is demanding what you want and what you have a right to. The young husband whose wife keeps her eyes shut during lovemaking has a right to something more. He married her in part because he thought that she would writhe in joy when he united his body with hers and thereby give unmistakable confirmation to his powers as a man. He has a right to such confirmation and ought to directly and vigorously demand it. In no uncertain terms he should tell his wife that he will settle for nothing less and that her shame and prudery are intolerable.

Similarly, the young wife who is getting no satisfaction out of intercourse should not be content with the gift of a book to her husband. She has a right to sexual satisfaction and she should demand that right. In the clearest possible terms she should tell her husband that so far he has been a failure as a lover and that she expects far more skillful passion from him—immediately. It is time that he begin to use her body the way it was intended to be used.

Unfortunately for the man in the one marriage and the woman in the other, "making demands" runs against what they have been taught that love is. In their family lives, they have learned that love means putting up with and going along with frustration and disappointment. One demonstrates love by being tolerant and not making demands. Love, in other words, means martyrdom, giving up one's own desires in order not to displease the other.

They have been taught what is not true. In fact, a love that is not passionate enough to demand the best from the other is not love at all.

But if the need for confrontation, conflict, and communication is especially obvious in the genital dimensions of a human relationship, it is in a way more simple when the subject is lovemaking. One is, after all, dealing with behavior that is relatively uncomplicated and with techniques that are relatively well known, at least in fantasy. Most men in their fantasy lives know exactly how to arouse their wives, but they are afraid to risk converting their fantasy into reality. Virtually every woman knows quite clearly and quite explicitly what it takes to make her husband feel supremely and ecstatically masculine, yet she is afraid to act on her knowledge for fear that her own defenses will be shattered permanently by such behavior. Communication and resolution are relatively easy where the problem is the need for progress in sexual adjustment. To say that the challenge is "relatively easy" is not to say that all that many people respond to it. It is simply to assert that the other problems of human intimacy are both more complex to describe and more difficult to resolve. There is both a fantasy and a folklore that men and women can fall back upon in providing sexual satisfaction for themselves and each other; there is much less folklore and almost no fantasy about how we adjust to intimacy with the person who is different from us—different not only in body but in personality. It is very unlikely that in marriage psychological conflicts can be worked out unless some basically satisfying modality of sexual adjustment has been achieved. If a husband and wife do not have fun with each other in bed, they will have neither the motivation nor the courage to tackle the more complex problems in a personality conflict. But being honest and blunt with each other about what is required for satisfactory intercourse is only the beginning—though a necessary one—for working out the ritual of conflict in the marriage.

Confrontation is not something distinct from the rhythm of taking and being taken in any human friendship. It is not a diversion from the process but a continuation and a furtherance of it. It can only occur when two people are confident enough of themselves and of their relationship to know that it can survive conflict and occasional acts of confrontation. But if this minimum confidence in the relationship does not exist and if conflict and confrontation cannot occur, then the two people who pretend to intimacy may continue to exist in some sort of physical or psychological juxtaposition, but friends and lovers they are not.

9

There are two kinds of loneliness that afflict human life. The first is the loneliness that comes from the human condition. It can be mitigated and alleviated but it cannot be eliminated. The other is the loneliness that we choose freely. It can always be conquered if we choose to do so.

We are, for weal or woe, consciously individuated creatures. No love, however permanent or however powerful, makes us more than finite. We may occasionally break through the boundaries of our finitude in moments of ecstasy. But these moments experienced in mystic contemplation or at the height of sexual arousal are fleeting, and we find ourselves all too quickly alone again, cut off, isolated. Genital love even at its most rewarding does not eliminate finitude though it can be a powerful motivation for temporarily achieving union. It alleviates, however transiently, the pain and isolation of finitude, and that is all that can be asked of it. Even the most ecstatic of experiences still leaves one lonely because it still leaves one finite. It is in these experiences that man feels most poignantly his hunger for the infinite. That there is an Infinite, incidentally, does not seem a matter for doubt during or immediately after moments of ecstasy. Such confidence in the Infinite is not, I think, exactly a "proof" that there is a Lover "out there" who will be able to end our loneliness. It rather reassures us of the existence of that love. It may well be the most important reassurance.

In addition to such existential loneliness, there is also the loneliness we freely choose. Even if man may not break completely with his finitude and isolation, his life is filled with opportunities to move beyond the barriers of individuation to find psychological and physical union with others. The pleasures and delights of life and love are obvious and demanding. Our bodies and our spirits are designed to seek union with others, but the design does not deprive us of our freedom. We can turn away from others; we can permit ourselves to be permanently rebuffed by them; we can lose our nerve, our courage, our imagination, our capacity for surprise. We can settle for a dull, monotonous, isolated, drab existence. We can do these things despite the primal thrust for union of body and spirit that is at the core of our personalities. To some extent, all of us choose this path of loneliness. One's giving and taking is always imperfect and inadequate. We are distracted, worried, anxious; and love is a very incomplete effort. What is important, however, is not perfection but persistence—a continuation of efforts to succumb to desire, to break out of fears, to become vigorous, challenging, surprising lovers. Even if their efforts seem to involve loss of dignity and propriety and leave them open to ridicule, lovers must persist.

Our existential loneliness is part of the human condition. Any celibate who thinks that if he had a spouse his life would have meaning and purpose and that he would be able to escape the finitude and imperfection that plague him is naive about both sexuality and meaning. How we interpret sexual experience is not at all dictated by the experiences themselves. Nor does sexuality remove the pains of isolation and individuation for very long. It does provide us with powerful motives and powerful rewards for not surrendering to isolation and withdrawing permanently behind the impenetrable barriers of loneliness. But a man whose life has no meaning before he finds a mate, who is mired down in his own distrust and suspicion, will find neither purpose nor cure for his loneliness amid the delights a woman's body offers. She is made to be enjoyed (as, indeed, a man is made to be enjoyed), but joy does not give faith and it does not heal fear. It may give a greater reason for faith and a more powerful drive against fear, but by itself pleasure is no cure for the sickness of spirit.

What sexuality does make possible—and in this respect the sexuality need not be genital—is affection and tenderness. And perhaps in the final analysis this is what women and men most need and most want in their lives. Orgasms are nice, but affection and tenderness are indispensable. A lover does indeed provide delight, but he also protects, provides care, and helps to avoid discouragement, weariness, and boredom. No lover can eliminate these things from his (or her) life unless he (or she) is willing to fight them; but in moments when the fight seems scarcely worth the effort, the lover can show that it is. It is precisely in these moments that human love is most rewarding, most pleasurable, and most important. Whoever loves and whatever be the nature of this love, if the lover knows when to say the kind word and to apply the gentle touch, when to laugh and smile, when to encourage and to show solicitude, when to sympathize with frustrations and to ridicule hesitancies, then the lover has immense power.

The need for affection of this kind is specifically human. It occurs only in creatures capable of reflection and who have devised symbols that give meaning to their behavior. But because affection is uniquely human, it becomes the indispensable prerequisite for human love. No matter how skilled the eroticism or genitality of lovers may be, if they do not make love in an atmosphere permeated by affection and tenderness, then their love will not be humanly satisfying. Man wants pleasure, of course, but he wants with it reassurance and comfort, and if these qualities are absent the pleasure really isn't that much fun. The most delightful lovemaking among married couples is precisely that which is explicitly designed to alleviate loneliness, discouragement, and weariness. It is then that love most effectively communicates to the other that he is worth something, that he is desired, admired, and loved. The wife comes to distract her husband from the worries of his work with herself and the martini pitcher. She is saying that however serious the work problems may be and however much he may be discouraged, it has nothing to do with his own goodness and desirability. She loves him and wants him no matter what happens, and she is willing to engage in "shameless" behavior to make it as clear as possible to him how much she wants him and how important he is to her no matter what else happens.

And a husband who gently calms his wife at the end of what was for her a nerve-racking, compulsive, and distracting day is telling her in effect that even if she feels she has failed to meet all of the multitudinous responsibilities that she could have coped with in the course of the day, she is still his and the source of constant delight to him not because of what she accomplished today but because of who she is. As the nightgown slips from her body, she knows not merely that she can give pleasure but also that she is a person who is cared for. That makes both the pleasure she gives and the pleasure received more intense.

Perhaps the reason for much of the infidelity that occurs in the early middle years of life is precisely that tenderness and affection have gone out of the marriage. It has become a series of obligations and responsibilities. Career (for one or for both), children, social life, political involvement, intellectual concerns—all of these use up time and energy, and while the two people still have intercourse with each other, it becomes more of a mechanical ritual than an act of reassurance and affection. *"INTERCOURSE"*

It is at just such times that a person most obviously needs affection and is most likely to attract it from others. Similarly, at such times affection offered or even available can become irresistible. One gets into an affair not so much for genital release (though that is surely to be had), not so much for erotic excitement (though that is certainly present), but so that one might experience a few moments of tenderness and reassurance. One may even know that such reassurance and affection are transient, shallow, and deceptive. Nonetheless, in times of loneliness and discouragement even shallow reassurance and transient affection will be eagerly accepted when nothing else is available.

In other instances, husband and wife withhold affection from each other not because they are thoughtless or distracted but because they deliberately intend to punish each other. The inevitable conflict between them is not faced but repressed; desire is converted into anger and delight into vindictiveness. All the slights, the insensitivities, the disappointments, and the frustrations build up and affection is refused precisely at the times when it is most obviously needed. Heaven help the other person if in desperation he turns to someone else for affection, because that provides even more grounds for punishment.

The vindictive withholding of affection (and one can concede one's body without offering affection) is one of the ugliest things a man or a woman can do. In the strict sense of the word, it is hateful. In the old days, Catholic women used to feel constrained to confess when they had refused their "marital duty." What they meant, of course, was that they had refused to have intercourse with their husbands, but the "marital duty," or indeed the duty of any love, goes far beyond physical union. What really ought to be confessed before God and men is the refusal to offer tenderness, affection, reassurance, and comfort to our lover at times when he or she most clearly needs it. There are times, of course, when people can be excused for not having intercourse, but there are no times, so long as there is anything left of the relationship, when they can be excused from tenderness and comfort.

It is man's loneliness and his need for affection that make possible those two difficult and pleasurable experiences between lovers, reconciliation and new beginnings. Not all conflict can be routinized; not all problems can be resolved. Confrontation may lead to a breakdown in the relationship, and fear may so impede communication that lovers become strangers. To begin again means to admit one's past mistakes, accept responsibility for one's failures, write off all the wasted time, and go back, as it were, to ground zero to begin again. Such a wiping clean of the slate, which involves forgiving both the other and oneself, is not an easy task. A married couple in their late thirties or early forties will be greatly humiliated to admit to each other that their genital life is dull and always has been. It will be tough for the man to concede that he has been inept and clumsy in his attempts to give pleasure to his wife. It will be hard for her to admit that part of the reason for his clumsiness has been her silence and another part of it has been that she long since gave up trying to be seductive. They must go back to the beginning and pretend that they are newlyweds or, perhaps more appropriately, that they are engaged in an illicit love affair. Indeed, by the standards of the routine to which their life together has sunk, any change will look like an illicit love affair. Each new beginning will not be easy, for it will mean that two people have learned from the mistakes that occurred in their relationship without holding these mistakes against each other. There are delights in reconciliation, of course, and a love affair that begins for the first time or anew at forty can be infinitely more pleasurable than one that begins at eighteen, for both lovers have much more experience, both physical and psychological, to bring to their affair. The past can be an asset as well as a liability, particularly if the lovers are able to develop a capacity to laugh at the grotesqueries of their past mistakes. They had better be able to laugh, because that is the only thing that will exorcise the anger and the humiliation of those mistakes.

It is the need for affection and reassurance that

is the most powerful motivation for beginning anew. Most lovers cannot or will not end their relationship unless it has become completely intolerable. There are too many things at stake. It is much better to stumble along in an unsatisfactory relationship than risk the public conflict, complication, and disgrace that would come from ending it. While extramarital interludes may provide temporary affection and reassurance, they tend to become unsatisfactory in the long run. One will find comfort and affection with one's spouse or probably not at all. Of course, there is a strong strain toward renewing affection because the couple have been lovers before, and are still, to some greater or lesser extent.

What has happened is that love and hatred have been powerfully intermixed in their relationship. The ambivalence that is involved in every intimacy is now both a serious problem and a last opportunity. The man and woman really do not like each other very much and have stored up all sorts of resentments. On the other hand, there are strong ties that unite them, and they can on occasion provide each other with both reassurance and pleasure.

In most marriages that have grown cool if not cold, there is in both people a latent desire to begin again, though, unfortunately, they have grown skilled in ignoring the cues that the other emits about the possibility of starting anew. What is required to begin a reconciliation is that when one person sees a tentative sign of affection and reassurance from the other, he or she should quickly respond with similar affection. There is, of course, considerable risk in either offering or responding to affection offered in a relationship that has become routine if not cool. In a way, it is an even bigger risk than beginning a love relationship, for now one knows all the things that can go wrong, and one also knows that if one attempts to renew a relationship and the other turns him down, it will make matters worse instead of better. Unfortunately, offers for renewal are frequently turned down. No one suspects that if such offers are firm enough, persistent enough, and imaginative enough, they will ultimately become irresistible in most cases.

A reconciliation involves winning a husband or wife all over again. It can be an exhilarating, fascinating, fun-filled experience. Indeed, any good marriage is a never-ending series of reconciliations. The more frequent the minor ones, the less need there will be to go through the pain of having a love relationship hit rock bottom before it begins to be reborn.

It frequently seems to those who are presented with an opportunity to begin again, to rebuild a relationship, that they are being asked to do something heroic and extraordinary. Winning each other all over again in the middle years of life seems ludicrous and absurd and simply not the thing to do. If, despite the evidence of realistic common sense, two people do begin anew, each of them may feel that what they are doing ought to be greatly rewarded. In a way they are correct. What they are doing is heroic and the rewards may very well be great, but any other course is the sheerest sort of folly. One either seeks reconciliation or settles down to a life of drab, affectionless routine in which there is no excitement, no tenderness, no affection, no reassurance. Our whole existence ought to be a constant refusal of such an alternative. No matter how much humiliation and forgiveness are involved, we must not choose loneliness.

10

Fidelity is part of every human friendship. It is the strain toward permanence and toward public commitment to permanence that is involved in any relationship beyond the most superficial. Fidelity is a longing for love that does not end.

Since every human relationship except the most transient has a sexual component to it, one can say that sexual fidelity ought to be a characteristic of all meaningful human relationships. The style of fidelity may vary from relationship to relationship. A man is faithful to another man who is his friend in a very different way than he is faithful to his wife. Similarly, he may be faithful to a woman who is a close friend in a very different way from the fidelity he exercises toward his wife. In this chapter we shall speak of fidelity between lovers who are permanently committed to one another with a special emphasis on genital fidelity. It should be clear that, as in so many other things, genital fidelity is merely a model and a symbol of a much more general aspect of human relationships.

The promise to be faithful to one's friend is by its very nature both permanent and public. A faithfulness that is secret is a peculiar kind of faithfulness indeed, because as long as it is secret one has the much easier option of going back on it. A man or a woman who intends to be faithful is eager to announce this fidelity to the whole community and to have the community ratify it. Faithfulness by its very nature seeks the public domain. Nor does faithfulness have any restrictions, limitations, or qualifications. When one pledges fidelity to a friend, he doesn't do it on a tentative basis or for a limited period of time or subject to an option for later renewal. Fidelity that is not aimed toward permanence is not fidelity at all.

I do not think that there can be much serious question that both public ratification and permanence are part of the notion of fidelity no matter what sort of relationship that fidelity characterizes. Having made this observation, let me note that the purpose of this chapter is not to make any judgment about such circumstances that might arise in a marriage when it might be concluded either that the promise of fidelity was never truly meant or that, for one reason or another, it may now no longer be considered binding. Neither do I propose to address myself to the question of whether a public and permanent commitment to another person may occur before it is solemnly ratified in a marriage ceremony. Hence, I will not speak of the question of divorce or the possibility of premarital sex. I refuse to address myself to these questions because they are beyond the scope of this book and because I think they can be addressed intelligently only after the material presented in this chapter is reflected upon.

It is interesting that the almost universally accepted definition of marital fidelity focuses on whether one engages in sexual activity outside of marriage. The faithful person is one who does not have intercourse outside of marriage. In no other context is fidelity defined in such narrow and negative terms. Indeed, normally the word conveys a highly positive connotation; but in marriage, fidelity merely means that one doesn't do certain things. It is at least possible that such a narrow and negative definition of marital fidelity has become widespread because it is much more difficult to follow the positive implications of the concept of fidelity in marriage than it is to stay out of someone else's bed.

Fidelity in any relationship is a permanent commitment to "reach out" for the other, a promise to persist in efforts to transcend the barriers and the distance that separate one from the other, a firm resolve to maintain effort in sustaining and developing the relationship no matter what difficulties and trials arise.

Genital fidelity, then, means that one is firmly committed to developing, enriching, and expanding the genital relationship with one's partner no matter how many frustrations, disappointments, and failures may intervene. The faithful lover is committed to developing his own skills, sensitivities, and capacities as a sexual being, particularly by learning through the "feedback" he receives from the other's response to him. He promises to give himself over to the physical and verbal dialogue that is required if his hesitant and tentative physical resources are to become firm, confident, and effective.

The faithful lover, then, engages in ongoing effort to improve the seductiveness of his erotic self-display. He constantly seeks to improve and refine his skills at bringing pleasure to the other. He develops his capacity for tenderness and especially his skill at combining tenderness with arousal. He arouses his partner in such a way that the weariness, discouragement, weakness, and fear that beset her or him are assuaged precisely in the process of responding to his (or her) sexual advances. *

Simultaneously, he strives ever more effectively to open up his own inner self, with all its fragility, vulnerability, and weaknesses, to the other so that the other may perceive his need for tenderness, affection, and gentleness, particularly when those qualities are communicated by the caress, the kiss, an embrace, a touch, a contact between warm and aroused bodies.

No one, be it noted, is born with such refined skills. While fantasy lives give general outlines, they do not provide detailed sets of instructions. The skills and sensitivities and capacities of being effective bed partners come only through practice, trial and error, through the ability to laugh at blunders, and, of course, from getting feedback from a partner. If a lover cannot persuade the one with whom he couples on the marriage bed to tell him what he is doing right and what wrong, then improvement is most unlikely. Fidelity means, then, that a lover asks for, indeed demands, such feedback; that it is done in such a way that the instructions from the other, be they in word or action, are a pleasure to give.

For a man to persist in this kind of fidelity is much more difficult than to turn away from the curvaceous body of a woman other than his wife when that body signals its availability to him. Rejecting the offer of a new body requires courage and strength of rather limited duration. Trying to improve one's capacity to bring pleasure to and obtain pleasure from a body that is next to one in bed every night is a challenge that never ends. *IMPORTANT!*

Similarly, a woman may have to push her resources to the limit to turn away from caresses that seem to almost set her on fire; but once she has turned away, she is not likely to have to turn away again from those hands if she has been definite in her rejection. The crisis was fierce but passing. Her husband's hands, however, are always present, capable indeed of bringing her great pleasure even though at times they may be clumsy and inept and occasionally totally lacking in attractiveness. Her commitment is not merely to permit her husband's hands to roam about her body but to guide them, help them, make them stronger and more confident. That is not a challenge of half an hour; it is the challenge of a lifetime.

Fidelity also means a commitment to increasing sensitivity to the other. First of all, the faithful lover has pledged himself to becoming ever more sophisticated in his understanding of the physiology of his genital partner. A man may know about women's physiology in general and still know nothing of his wife's. And unless fidelity means for him the responsibility of tenderly and gently exploring her body and her responses to that exploration, he will never know. That a very considerable number of men have only the most remote notions of the physiological responses of women and practically no notion at all of the particular responses of their wives indicates how little this dictate of fidelity is honored.

In our culture it is assumed that a man's physiological response is more obvious than a woman's. Hence, a wife may feel that she does indeed understand the physiology of her husband and there is no further need to explore his body. What he is looking for is obvious enough, and there is no need for subtlety or nuance or delicacy in what she does. But in fact the flesh and the nervous system of a man are as delicate and responsive as they are in a woman. There is an infinite variety of shadings and nuances in what a woman can do to the body of a man. When either partner thinks there is nothing more to be learned, then the commitment to growth and self-transcendence in a genital relationship is in trouble.

But fidelity also implies the desire to grow in understanding of the psychosexual needs and dispositions of the partner. The one who is loved is more than a collection of sexual organs, primary and secondary, to be stimulated. He or she also possesses a rich, complex fantasy life, and the lover wishes to penetrate into this fantasy life because the lover seeks more knowledge and because the fantasy life is the raw material for maintaining surprise and wonder in lovemaking.

The faithful lover learns how to read the defense mechanisms of his genital partner with skills like that with which the professional quarterback reads the defensive secondary. For, just as in football, the defenses change as the circumstances change, so in lovemaking the moods, the fears, the hopes, the frustrations of a given situation may make for a rather different set of defense mechanisms than the ones that existed last night or may exist tomorrow night. Similarly, the faithful lover does all in his power to increase his sensitivity to the cues that his beloved emits, indicating the need for tenderness and affection. He works hard to learn how to overcome the other's reluctance to talk about what happens when the last garment is laid aside and the erectile tissues begin to prepare for union.

Finally, the faithful lover strives to become gracious in the techniques of providing the other with the needed feedback in such a way as to enhance rather than weaken fundamental self-esteem as a sexual person and as a genital partner. To inform, instruct, correct, lead in a way that enhances self-esteem is no easy task. It requires delicacy, tact, discretion, and also the ability to ultimately say exactly what one means. No one knows naturally how to communicate with others in such a fashion, particularly when the subject is as sensitive and primordial as lovemaking; and yet, unless man and woman are committed to growing in such skills and helping each other to grow, it is not clear that their marriage ought to be described as a faithful one.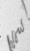

The use I have made of the notion of fidelity in this chapter seems strange only because we have been willing to accept a narrow, negative definition of the term. I am arguing that fidelity means only in a secondary and relatively unimportant way that we do not commit adultery. In a primary and positive way it means that married lovers are committed to developing a pleasurable genital relationship that has within it the capacity for ever more development no matter how many obstacles or difficulties or frustrations or disappointments may be encountered. One might add that fidelity seems almost necessarily to involve a commitment on the part of lovers that they will never stop laughing at their mistakes, ineptitudes, and blunders; for if they cannot sustain their capacity for laughter, it is to be feared that laughter's cynical surrogate, ridicule, will intervene. Laughter can unite lovers psychologically, first, and then physically; ridicule divides, separates, and isolates.

What has been described in this chapter is merely genital fidelity: the commitment to increasing both one's own pleasure and the pleasure of the spouse. Of course, genital fidelity is only part of the more total human fidelity that should permeate the whole marriage relationship. However critical a symbol it may be of the marriage relationship, it is subsidiary to the wider meaning of fidelity in marriage, as in any friendship. Fidelity in this broader sense means the permanent, public, solemn, and irrevocable commitment to dedicate one's life to bringing out the best in both one's partner and oneself. It is most unlikely that a man and woman will be able to do this unless there is a strong commitment to increasing the amount of enjoyment that occurs in sexual relations. On the other hand, if there is not a relationship in which two people are committed to a whole life of challenging the best that is in each other, then it is not likely that the union of sex organs will continue to be very enjoyable.

It is interesting to observe that many married people experience great feelings of guilt when they sleep with someone else but relatively little feeling of guilt when they allow the nightly or thrice-weekly romp on the marriage bed to become dull and routine. The husband will torment himself about a transient affair with a woman at work or a brief fling when he is away at a convention. These are acts of infidelity, but it will never occur to him that a continuing infidelity occurs when he acquiesces in the static and stagnant genital relationship with his wife.

Similarly, a woman will torment herself (and frequently her confessor) endlessly about an episode of infidelity when she seduces or permits herself to be seduced by the handsome, virile man across the street one day when his wife and her husband are away somewhere else. She will not permit herself even the slightest consideration of the possibility that there may have been mitigating circumstances, and she would be horrified at the suggestion that a basic infidelity permeates the whole relationship with her husband because she has permitted it to become dissatisfying and uninteresting. The human race continues to strain at the gnat and swallow the camel.

Fidelity, then, means a refusal to give up on a relationship. Genital fidelity means the refusal to give up on the possibility of enhancing the excitements and the satisfactions available in the union between a male and a female body. Marital fidelity, in the most general sense, means that a husband and wife refuse to give up on their relationship until every last possible effort has been expended.

Infidelity is not the same thing as adultery, at least in its primary meaning. Infidelity means quitting, giving up on any aspect of a relationship when there are still possibilities remaining. Adultery frequently may be the result of this primordial infidelity, and it may also contribute to an infidelity that is spreading through a relationship like a cancer; but as long as there is a commitment to continue efforts to try to expand and to grow, to be a better, more generous, and more effective lover, then adultery does not of itself destroy the primary fidelity of a genital relationship. It is an unfortunate and ugly incident, but it does not necessarily revoke a primary commitment.

Fidelity assumes that the basic evaluation of the other, which led to the original commitment, was a correct one; it may have been naive or incomplete, but it was a commitment that saw something valuable and admirable in the other. The other was initially perceived as fun to be with, fun to look at in the nude, challenging to go to bed with, and exciting enough to want to spend a lifetime with. The frustrations, disappointments, and disillusionments that have intervened since that initial commitment cannot help but call it into question. Fidelity persists in believing that the original valuation was correct and that it would be a mistake to abandon without further effort the struggle to achieve the good things that the original commitment promised.

Essential to fidelity is gentleness. We are all of us fragile, uncertain, vulnerable, insecure, hesitant people. The more we act as though we are not, the more we reveal our own weakness. Only the strong person can admit that he is weak. There are few human relationships and few marriages that will not notably improve when the gentleness level in the relationship is increased.

If what happens in the marriage bed is not pervaded by gentleness, it is likely to be both unsatisfying and infrequent. Sophisticated lovers know that in the bedroom or anywhere else gentleness has incredible erotic power. A kiss at the nape of the neck, a contact of two hands, an arm around the waist, tentative pressure of a knee against a thigh, fingers brushing lightly and quickly across a breast— all of these gentle actions have much more powerful erotic impact than do the acrobatics and gymnastics of the sex manuals performed without gentleness. Fidelity, then, is persistent, dauntless, implacable when need be, challenging when challenge is called for, and, in the midst of everything, always gentle.

The most basic reason for lack of sexual satisfaction is neither cognitive nor psychological; it is rather existential. Many people lack the basic information, or at least the detailed information, to be adequate sexual partners. Many more—probably most— have psychological hang-ups that stand in the way of using the information they do have. Information can be obtained and psychological problems can be lessened by competent therapy. But unless they are willing to believe that they are lovable and attractive as human beings and that the risk of vulnerability is underwritten by a fundamentally gracious cosmos, their sex lives are not going to be especially rewarding.

A man may watch a full-color movie (of the sort currently being used in sex education) of a man bringing a woman to full climax with his hand. Such a movie may well impart potentially useful information and it will certainly arouse him erotically, but it will not persuade him that he is either a skillful lover or an attractive man unless his wife's attitude toward him leaves little doubt about it.

Similarly, a woman may digest all the suggestions of *The Sensuous Woman* and never consider using any of them in bed unless she is convinced that her husband loves her and finds her irresistible as a woman.

With few exceptions, lovers enter sexual relationships with very uncertain faith in their own attractiveness and competency. Those who behave most confidently are usually the most insecure. They need both the faith that they can take risks and the response of a lover whose desire is so apparent that it creates desirability. Neither information nor therapy— however useful and appropriate they may be—can in itself persuade one to take the risks of exposed vulnerability in a complete sexual relationship. Faith in the possibility of fidelity (as it has been described in this chapter) is essential if one is to go beyond information and therapy to the great adventure of sexual love.

Thus a spouse must face the fact that no matter how confident the other may seem, he (or she) is not really confident at all, and the absolutely essential prerequisite of sexual growth is to build up the other's confidence in his (or her) own sexuality. To the extent that one can persuade the partner that he (or she) is "good in bed"—or in any other dimension of the marriage—will the partner in fact become "good" there.

Fidelity means dedicating one's life to creating an irresistible lover out of a very human partner. The faithful man knows that unless his wife is convinced that it is her erotic appeal rather than his "needs" that turns him on whenever he is with her, she will not be much of a "playmate," and their marriage will be listless and dull. His conviction about her eroticism makes it possible for her to be erotic.

And the faithful woman knows that her husband will be clumsy and inept unless she conveys to him that she has no choice but to melt in his presence, that she desperately craves to feel his body inside of hers. Only then will he have enough confidence in his manhood to be the kind of man that can in fact send her into paroxysms of pleasure. In lovemaking you get what you earn.

Essential to creating an irresistible lover for oneself is knowing what to see. Every lover is physically capable of arousing a partner if only because the organs are meant to complement. Nor are there any partners so inept that there do not exist in them the faint stirrings of eroticism. They must then choose to "see" that which is attractive and erotic and ignore that which is still and awkward. If one chooses to invest the other with eroticism and gently helps to develop it, one has in fact yielded to the other's attractiveness. By selecting those aspects of behavior and person that can be developed into extreme eroticism, and by responding to such aspects, the lover makes it possible for them to be developed. By ignoring or brushing aside fears and hesitancies it is thus made possible for them to diminish. By selective perceptions a lover can make another what that partner is capable of becoming.

Of course, just the opposite can be done by choosing to ignore the first tentative movements of adult genitality and concentrating on the mistakes, the stiffness, the ridiculous false starts. Such a response drives the other back into his shell—freeing the one from the obligation to run the risks of growth.

And that is the essence of infidelity.

Part of the promise of fidelity, it seems to me, is the commitment to maintain physical attractiveness in keeping with one's age. Presumably, this means that the "overweight and out-of-shape" condition of most middle-class Americans is in some sense a violation of such a commitment. A man or a woman who permits the body to become flabby and fat is saying in effect that there is no need to maintain a sexually attractive appearance. There are two possible reasons for such a decision. Either it is a means of keeping the lover at bay or it is a means of punishing oneself for sexual frustration and inadequacy. In either case, the body is being used as a barrier and not as a means of communication.

I will confess to being shocked at the number of young people still in their twenties who will pay large sums of money each year for clothes and cosmetics but are apparently willing to distort their bodies by eating too much and not exercising enough.

And the claim that being overweight has nothing to do with sexual fears and frustrations ought to be perceived as patently absurd in an era as informed on the teachings of Dr. Freud as ours claims to be.

In the entire range of the components of a marriage, what fidelity means is that one commits oneself never to wait for the other to take the initiative to heal a separation and never to reject the other's initiative no matter how awkward or inarticulate that initiative may be.

Fidelity means that when a woman wakes in the middle of the night from a frightening dream and feels lonely and worthless and afraid, she does not hesitate to reach for her husband, knowing that he has the strength, confidence, and tenderness to exorcise her primordial fears. It means she knows that not to seek his consolation under such circumstances would be infidelity, because it would mean that she is not willing to share with him her most intimate feelings of weakness.

Similarly, fidelity means that at the end of a frustrating, discouraging humiliating day a husband knows that he can and must give the signals to his wife by which she will know that he needs an encounter with a primal, life-giving earth mother who can smother his feelings of inadequacy with the delights of her flesh. Not to turn to her for comfort under such circumstances is also infidelity, because it means that he is not willing to share with her his most intimate weakness.

In every faithful relationship, there are turning points: decisive occasions when the whole tone and ambiance of the relationship are transformed. But there will be one point that is crucial because it points the way to all the others. Married couples whose genital interaction is satisfying emphasize that there was a time when their lovemaking went through a drastic transformation, when they were able stimultaneously to shed their fears, their inhibitions, their uncertainties, and confusions. Usually, such an event occurred when they found themselves saying and doing things that they never thought they could be able to say and do and couldn't quite believe in fact that they had taken the drastic risk that seemed to be involved. Once they crossed such a sexual Rubicon, everything that went before looked in retrospect like foolishness. Unfortunately, such decisive ventures into the land of sexual pleasure never happen in many marriages—though many times they *almost* happen. At the last moment, both man and woman lose their nerve.

A man may have many distractions and problems on his mind. He may have a whole host of critical responsibilities that must be thought about and acted upon; but when he senses that his wife is possessed by a feeling of worthlessness as a woman, he must mobilize all his resources as a man to convince her that she is wrong. Not a single sexually sensitive part of her body should remain untouched by his fiercely roaming fingers or lips. If he cannot restore her faith in her womanhood under such circumstances, he is worthless as a husband, no matter how many fur coats he may buy for her.

When a woman sees that her husband is battered and harried, discouraged and beaten, nothing is more important in her life than to comfort and caress him. His weary head must be pressed against her and her hands must blot out all the aches and pains of his existence. When she is finished loving him, life once again will be eminently worth living, if only because he knows that whatever else he may lose, she will always be there.

Such occasions of weakness and vulnerability are critically important in a marriage precisely because there are times when a lover has immense power over his (or her) mate. The power will be used either to break into a previously unexplored area of the other's selfhood to draw the lovers closer to one another, or it will be used to demolish an already bruised and fragile ego. It is a melancholy reflection on the state of contemporary American marriages to suspect that the latter is a much more frequent occurrence than the former.

But the faithful lover is constantly sensitive to the possibility that the other may be saying in word or deed, "Please, please love me *now*." For when that message is sent, the opportunity for growth in both physical love and personal pleasure is very great indeed. To miss such an opportunity is infidelity of the worst sort.

I take it that when fidelity is so understood, it is naturally an admirable characteristic. Despite the pseudosophistication of some of the sex literature, few people really admire infidelity. The playboy and the playmate may look attractive in the shallow glitter of Mr. Hefner's journal, but few would want to spend too much time with either of these characters. In fact, the whole appeal of the *Playboy* philosophy is that it promises quick pleasure without having to be involved with the rather dull pasteboard people who provide it. The ambiguity of fidelity consists in the fact that it is both admirable and difficult, both something to be valued highly and something that is very difficult to practice because it demands so much of our resources.

The struggle for fidelity—as that quality has been defined in this chapter—is difficult; but it is also pleasurable, indeed, immensely so. When two people are trying to grow in their mutual lovemaking, a psychological tone develops in their relationship that greatly enhances their attractiveness to each other. The fact of their joint effort is a partial guarantee of its success, precisely because the joy of their common quest makes them more pleasurable—

in the sense both of being able to give and of being able to receive pleasure—to one another. They love one another more because there is more to love.

✻Sleeping with someone else is always a radical possibility because they always have the physical capacity of coupling with anyone, but however powerful a transient inclination to do so may be, they are still likely to confine their genital activity to the marriage bed. With no other potential partner do they share the exquisite pain and the exquisite joy of the quest for fidelity.￼Other partners may *look* more attractive for a few moments or a few days, but the faithful lover knows that his (or her) permanent partner is more attractive because it took a long time to develop the acute sensitivity to the possibilities of pleasure that can be found in a faithful relationship.￼Familiarity breeds contempt only for those who have stopped growing. For faithful lovers, it breeds both heightened pleasure and even heightened mystery.

Can the Christian symbol system throw any light on the ambiguity of fidelity? Can it ensure that this admirable but painful human characteristic is possible? It seems to me that these are the pertinent questions that we must ask. Whether premarital or extramarital sex is sinful is not nearly so important as whether Christianity can sustain the positive demands of faithfulness. If it can, then the question of sex outside of marriage can be answered within a religious context. If it cannot, then the church is simply one more ethical or moral lawgiver with nothing new or unique to add to human customs.

The reason why we Christians are faithful in our relationships to one another is that Yahweh is faithful to us. In that implacable assertion in the book of Exodus, "I am Yahweh your God," he made it perfectly clear that no matter what we did as his people, he would still be our God. And in the sexual imagery of Hosea, Jeremiah, and Ezekiel, Yahweh emphasized that even though we whore with false gods, he will not seek another people. We might turn our backs on him; he will never turn his back on us. We might be unfaithful; he will never be unfaithful. The Good News that Jesus brought was in effect a renewal of that covenant. The cross and the resurrection were a new covenant precisely because they promised in a deeper and richer way Yahweh's fidelity. The Eucharist has frequently been compared to a wedding banquet precisely because it is a celebration of Yahweh's fidelity to his bride, the church. Christians are faithful to one another in all their relatioships because Yahweh's fidelity gives them the confidence that their own fidelity requires and because they understand that their fidelity is an exercise in their vocation of manifesting Yahweh's love to the world. When a Christian husband and wife are faithful to one another in the way I have described in this chapter, they are manifesting Yahweh's love to the world.

It is to be presumed that most married couples do not view the art of sexual intercourse as a reflection of Yahweh's fidelity, for after all it occurs in the privacy of their bedroom with the door closed and the lights dim. How could they possibly believe that improving their skills at bringing each other pleasure reflects God's implacable commitment to his people?

They don't think of these things, in all likelihood, because nobody has ever suggested to them that the quality of their love—of which sexual intercourse is, of course, at the very center—is the most effective way they have of revealing God's love to the rest of the world. To the extent that a man and woman have settled for a static and dull genital relationship, they have settled for a marriage that is a very inadequate reflection of God's love for mankind. And to the extent that they are committed to improving the surprise and pleasure, the excitement, the challenge of what goes on between the sheets, then they are reflecting God's commitment to his people.

It seems to me that this is the only fundamentally meaningful observation that Christianity can make on the subject of premarital or extramarital sex. We Christians are faithful to one another in all our relationships and especially in our marriages, because that is the way we reflect God's love for us. There may be social, psychological, philosophical, psychiatric, and legal arguments in favor of fidelity. I am not sure how effective these arguments are when the temptation to adultery is almost overwhelming. Perhaps the Christian perspective that I have sketched in this chapter is no more effective, but it seems to me that it is the one that is uniquely ours and the only one that we should spend much time emphasizing.

When I have made this argument, people have said to me, "Young people don't accept such an ideal." I am not sure how many young people would in fact reject the ideal of fidelity when it is described in the positive fashion I have attempted in this chapter, but if young people are so devoid of sensibility that they cannot appreciate the natural admirability of fidelity, then so much the worse for them, for they are dull and unperceptive. And if they do not believe that it is appropriate for Christians to reflect in their relationships the implacable fidelity of Yahweh to us, then, once again, so much the worse for them, because they are not Christians and they do not understand the wonder and joy of the Christian message.

My point is that we must begin with the fundamental Christian symbols if we are to make a unique contribution to the problem of human fidelity. If those to whom we are talking do not accept the Christian symbol system, if they are unwilling to believe in God's overwhelming fidelity toward us as manifested in his son Jesus, then religious dialogue between them and us is not possible. One does not begin the dialogue, in other words, by talking about premarital sex. Nor does one begin by talking about fidelity even in the positive sense I have used in this chapter. One begins by talking about God's fidelity to us and then by suggesting that such fidelity gives us both the strength and the motivation we need for the admirable but extraordinarily difficult human quality of faithfulness.

We have no reason to apologize for the ideal of Christian fidelity, be it the fidelity of a genital relationship or of any kind of human relationship. Fidelity is naturally admirable; the ideal of fidelity that reflects God's fidelity to us is religiously sensitive and inspiring. That many people will not accept the ideal does not mean that it is inadequate; it is not that it has, as G. K. Chesterton suggested in another context, "been tried and found wanting," but found hard and not tried.

If there is no reason to apologize for the ideal of Christian fidelity, there are plenty of reasons for apologizing for the narrow, negative, physiological definition that we have permitted to become identified with fidelity. It is time that we made it clear to all concerned that we will simply have no part in conversations that begin with, "What's wrong, after all, with premarital intercourse?" From our point of view, the conversation should begin with, "What's wrong with people who are not able to grow in pleasure and satisfaction, in giving and receiving in marital intercourse?"

11

Human sexuality is a burden, a burden as heavy as life itself. Conflict, loneliness, the need for wonder and surprise—all of these are part of the agony of the human condition. Humans can get much more satisfaction out of their sex lives than animals, but they have to work at it much harder. An animal does not need courage; he does not need to take risks; he merely does what his instincts tell him to do. Humans must have both courage and faith.

The young man whose passive wife closes her eyes when he is doing to her the things a man should be doing to a woman ought to be possessed by outraged fury. He ought to shake her angrily until her eyes open wide and shout, "Damn you! Look at me when I play with you!" Such a cry is as natural, as normal, and as inevitable as a cry of pain after one touches a hot stove. Those closed eyes and that limp, passive body give a devastating, if unintentional, rejection. And yet, to give voice to that cry of anger requires bravery. It is perhaps easier, if frustrating, to accept her prudery and shame.

Similarly, the young woman whose husband is a timid and disappointing lover is scarcely being very effective when she buys him a book. She should face him with withering scorn and demand, "Don't you know anything about how to seduce a woman?" Again, the cry of anger and pain flows naturally from the depths of the woman's person, and it may humiliate and enrage her husband, but in these circumstances it will be curative. Drift, resentment, frustration require little courage; curative anger requires much.

The courage required for a demand of sexual response is great, but it covers only one situation, albeit a very important one. The courage to face the constant tensions, frictions, and conflict of a life of intimacy is even more difficult, because it is not a courage that demands great anger in one situation but rather great persistence in all situations. We can be very brave for short periods of time, but constant bravery is wearisome.

It also takes courage to emit those small cues and signals that say to the other, "Please care for me—now. I desperately need reassurance and affection." It takes equal courage to live a life that is always sensitive to the possibility that such cues are being emitted. Only the brave can permit others to see them as they really are. We are afraid to stand naked physically in the presence of another because we are so vulnerable stripped. We can be ridiculed, baited, hurt. We are even more afraid to be psychically vulnerable in the presence of the other. If he knows us as we really are, how can he help but share the disgust we feel for ourselves? About all one can say to a lover who is seeking the courage for physical and psychological self-revelation is that just as the other's body and person delight you rather than disgust you, so, incredible as it may seem, your body and your spirit are not only adequate to him but a source of constant fascination and joy. But the battle between courage and shame is an unending one, and the victories of courage are both difficult to wage and barely won.

We can say about love what was said of the military history of Great Britain, that all battles were lost except the last one. It doesn't matter whether courage triumphs over shame by a slight margin; what matters is that it does in fact triumph.

But something more is required to sustain wonder, courage, capacity for growth, openness, the ability to deal with conflict, loneliness, and the imperfection of all human effort. And that is faith. Without faith both courage and love become impossible. I use the word "faith" in its most primordial sense. It is the conviction that despite distraction, discouragement, disappointment, failure, disillusionment, and frustration, it is still worth the effort to try to love and to be loved. Faith in this sense is a fully conscious commitment to the idea that life has worth and purpose and value. If one does not believe in the value of human life and the dignity of human effort, then one will simply not have the courage it takes to keep alive wonder and surprise, to engage in conflict and its resolution, to give and receive affection in a love relationship. The faith I have described is prereligious in the sense that we experience it at the core of our being before we use religious symbols to give expression to such a fundamental assurance of our own value and worth. Our religious symbols and myths, as Schubert Ogden has pointed out, are merely ways of re-presenting and reassuring us of this basic worth that is at the very core of the structure of our existence and awareness. Some religious symbols are more effective than others at re-presenting this primal assurance, and, of course, no religious symbol is so effective that we cannot turn away from that basic assurance and lead lives of grim, monotonous despair. All too many people assert religious symbols but live lives that give every evidence that the symbol is not taken too seriously as a way of viewing the world.

Schubert Ogden (*The Reality of God and Other Essays*, New York: Harper & Row, 1966, p. 116) has argued that there are two fundamental presuppositions to religious commitment:

> First, that life as we live it is somehow of ultimate worth; and, second, that it is possible to understand our selves and the world in their relation to totality so that this assurance of life's worth may be reasonably affirmed. Therefore, the criterion for assessing the truth of myths may be formulated as follows: *mythical assertions are true insofar as they so explicate our unforfeitable assurance that life is worthwhile that the understanding of faith they represent cannot be falsified by the essential conditions of life itself.*

The question, then, we must ask about our religious symbols is that when we "put them on" and view the world from their perspective, does this perspective reinforce our own fundamental self-assurance? And does it also enable us to interpret and to cope with the ambiguities of our existence? Those of us who are Christians must ask ourselves what the core of those symbols sheds on the ambiguities, the strains, the conflicts, the tensions, the demands of human love.

The central symbol of Christianity is the combination of the cross and resurrection. Jesus who died
now lives. How can that symbol possibly shed any
light on the complexities and ambiguities of human
sexual relationships?

I am afraid that one must say that it ought to be
obvious how the cross and resurrection are pertinent
to human sexuality. That it is not obvious comments
not on the ineffectiveness of the symbol but on our
own prudery and fear. The Christians of early Rome,
who transferred the pagan spring fertility rite of
plunging the candle into water, had no such difficulties. They knew that the lighted candle represented
the penis and that water represented a vagina and a
womb; and they knew, too, that their pagan friends
and neighbors performed this rite in order to guarantee the fertility of their fields, their animals, and
their wives. The early Christians thought that when
Christ rose from the dead, he consummated his union with his bride, the church. If the resurrection
looked like a sexual symbol then and does not look
like one to us, the reason, perhaps, is that they had a
much clearer realization than we do that life presumes fertility.

The cross and resurrection in their very core
mean to us that life triumphs over death, but that we
must die first. New life comes from being reborn, not
from escaping the necessity and the pain of death.
When we put on this cross-resurrection symbol we
are then able to see that each new conflict, each new
risk, each new thrust against loneliness is a death
that we must endure if we have hope to live anew.
The young lover must give death to his fears if he is
to shout at his wife that she should open her eyes
and look at him. But unless he is willing to die that
death, he will never experience the resurrection that

a sexually responsive wife would make possible. Similarly, the young wife who must take her husband's hand and firmly guide it must die a thousand deaths to her shame and prudery. But there is no escaping from this death if she wishes to have a new life of sexual arousal and satisfaction.

The middle-aged couple who tentatively and awkwardly begin to exchange tenderness and affection as a prelude to beginning their love affair all over again, or perhaps starting it for the first time, must go through the anguish of the damned (or something like it) to put aside the hurts and the resentments and the bitterness of the past. Only by dying to the mistakes and anger of the past can they expect to rise to a new life of affection and pleasure.

Everyone must die to the prudery and shame that make them shy and awkward if they are going to rise to a new life in which erotic self-display surrounds them with an ambiance of wonder and surprise. The woman approaching her husband with her nakedness covered only by a martini pitcher must die to the humiliating possibility that her husband won't be interested and will attempt to brush her off. The new dimension of sexual pleasure that her surprise can make possible will only in fact be a form of resurrection if she is determined to cope with a brush-off by telling him that either he instantaneously remove his clothes and make love to her or she will pour the martinis over his head and call a divorce lawyer.

A healthy genital relationship is one in which the two partners are engaged in the ongoing process of attracting and luring one another to bed. The conquest is never so complete, the surrender never so definitive that it need not be repeated. When the lover ceases to be a challenge, when he yields his body for pleasure with no effort on the partner's part, the game becomes uninteresting. Similarly, when a lover is permitted to take pleasure without having to lure, then the response is perfunctory, given almost as though something else were on the partner's mind. Genitality without mutual luring loses most of its eroticism; it becomes passionless passion.

When a man never sees a look of anticipation and invitation in his woman's eyes, and when she never feels his hand squeeze her thigh as she sits next to him in the car or pat her bottom as she climbs the steps ahead of him, their relationship has become dull and routine. Yet the necessity of winning one's partner over and over again is wearying. A comfortable, unexciting routine requires less effort, and it provides much less payoff.

The surprise component of sex has as its principal purpose the arousal of the other so that in his excitement he will pursue us. So, too, with Yahweh's intervention in human events. He surprises us in order that he might attract us. He excites us so that we might be drawn out of our mundane lives and pursue him. The Hound of Heaven image works both ways: God pursues us by attracting us to pursue him. But then that is the way every passionate lover acts.

Our Greek philosophy pictures God for us as the "unmoved mover." Our dull, dry catechetics has described him as a dispassionate judge who is sufficient unto himself and does not need us. But contemporary process theology, reflecting the Scriptures, describes him as a "tender companion" (to use Alfred North Whitehead's term) who attracts us to follow along with him by his gentle and seductive lures.

When a man and a woman practice their mutual wiles on one another they are imitating the way God works on us; and to the extent that these wiles draw them both out of their mundane narrowness, they are literally cooperating with God's gentle seductions. The more the lover excites the partner into a frenzy of passion, the more godlike he is. This is not merely exaggerated rhetoric; if we take the scriptural imagery seriously—and we must—it is literal truth.

A wife who passively accepts her husband's advances and never takes the initiative and who is "uninterested" in sex may think she is a dutiful woman and even something of a martyr. In fact she is not only dull and somewhat frigid, she has repressed the spark of divinity that abides in her female body. And the husband who "leaves his wife alone" except when the demand for tension release is irresistible may think he is a kind and considerate mate; but unless he can make his wife's body writhe in joy and her voice shout with uncontrolled pleasure, he is a failure as a man and is false to the power of the divinity that lurks in his body.

It is a mistake to think that God's love for us is the mild, circumspect *agape*, a bloodless, "nice" affection from which all passion has been drained. The God of the Testaments, New and Old, is not a "nice" God at all but a lover consumed with *eros*. It is disgraceful for his followers to mate with each other in any but the most fervent, erotic way. The greater the pleasure that man and woman give to each other—in bed and in every dimension of their relationship—the more is God present with them.

Does the cross-resurrection symbolism really apply to these events? Or is it merely an almost blasphemous distortion of the Jesus myth to say that the cross and resurrection give meaning and purpose to the anguish and ecstasy of human sexual encounter? One is forced to reply that if the cross-resurrection symbolism does not apply to such poignant and frequent human situations, it is not much good. But of course it does apply, for it tells us in the most dramatic religious terms possible that human growth comes through death and rebirth, and that it is safe to take the risk of dying because God has guaranteed us rebirth. If man need not fear the death that comes at the end of life, he surely need not fear the death of fear, uncertainty, and anxiety, which are a part of every important interpersonal encounter in his life.

I am not suggesting that the cross-resurrection symbol is the only religious symbol that says life is worth living. Neither would I wish to argue that it is necessarily the most powerful (though my own personal convictions would affirm its supreme power). I am merely suggesting that such arguments are foolish. The cross-resurrection symbol, which is at the core of the religious belief of every Christian, is readily available to Christians as an antidote to the fear and the suspicion that stand in the way of love.

Or to put the matter more graphically: When two naked lovers stand in each other's presence in that basic, fear-filled, and delight-filled human encounter, they are, if they are Christians, symbolically clad in the cross and the resurrection of Jesus. And if they are willing to look at each other and at themselves through the powerful light that that symbol sheds, they become far more attractive than they would be without it, because the symbol tells them that it is all right to take risks. Their Christian commitment assures them that they need not be afraid of the deaths they are going to have to die if their love is to continue and to grow. Those deaths are but a prelude to new life.

"Putting on" the symbols of the cross and resurrection of Jesus ought to make a man and woman far more sexy than putting on black lace underwear (though there's nothing wrong with that either). If the cross and resurrection do not make us more sexually attractive, that is not Jesus's fault. It's ours.

Part Two

LOVE AND
P L A Y

AUTHOR'S NOTE ON LOVE AND PLAY

The ten chapters that make up this essay are an argument for a sustained commitment in the sexual union, or, to use the old phrase, for permanency in marriage. But if I argue for something old, the arguments I use in support of it are, I think, rather new. For I shall contend in this essay that playfulness can occur in human relationships, and in particular the sexual relationship, only in an environment created by permanent commitment. Instead of conceding to my adversaries—as most of those who write in the Christian context do—that playfulness and variety are antithetical to the serious business of marriage, I shall argue that authentic playfulness and variety will occur only when there is a strong, sustained commitment between playmates. More than that, I also suggest that given the immense demands placed on the marital relationship today, it will either be playful or it will be considerably less than successful. If sex is not play, it may not be anything at all except occasions for periodic tension release. If marital sex is not playful, then the whole marriage relationship, which is symbolized, reinforced, underwritten, and manifested in its sexual dimension, is not viable. An oppressively close relationship such as marital intimacy is either playful or it is intolerable.

The argument is a novel one, I think. It will offend those libertarians who find marital fidelity and permanency a drag. It will also offend that far larger group of human beings who, caught in the grip of the puritan temptation, believe that marriage and sex are far too serious, far too important, and involve far too many responsibilities to allow anything as childish and frivolous as play to enter into the equation. Both groups bear a common assumption: Marriage is one thing and play is something else. The one group considers it to be axiomatic that "good" sex (by which they mean "fun" sex) occurs usually only outside marriage. The second group believes that there is no room in marriage for playful sex. My contention is that they are both wrong. "Good" (fun) sex can only be sustained in a context of a long-term commitment to one's partner, and "good" (moral) sex in marriage can grow only when playfulness characterizes all the dimensions of the intimacy between husband and wife. My argument will not be easily accepted by either side.

There are three basic assumptions that underpin this essay. The first is that it is necessary for those Christians who reflect on the meaning of human sexuality to temporarily bracket such questions as pre-, extra-, and comarital sexuality, as well as birth control, divorce, and abortion. These are by no means unimportant issues, but they can only be answered effectively when one has thought through once again what illumination the Christian symbol system can

shed on the ambiguity of human sexuality, and what
sense of direction it can provide for those who seek
to transcend the ambiguities in which they currently
find themselves. The resources of theology, philosophy, psychology, and sociology must be brought to
bear on the dilemmas of human sexuality so that we
can understand better the anguish, the poignance,
and the ambiguity of contemporary sexual relationships. We must determine whether any insight, any
understanding, can be gained from the Christian
symbol system as humankind attempts to cope with
these dilemmas.

Secondly, I assume as my principal concern the
dilemmas and ambiguities experienced by those who
are more or less permanently committed to one
another. Despite all the publicity given to alternative
sexual forms, most human sex, in fact, still occurs
between one man and one woman who have come
together in a familial relationship. There is absolutely
no reason to think that the situation will change. On
grounds of physical and social convenience, if for no
other reason, the family is likely to survive. For most
people the major problem is not extramarital or
premarital or comarital sex but marital sex. A sexual
theory that begins with deviations from the normal
(I mean here, "that which is most frequent") will not
be applicable to most human beings; and if it is not
applicable to most humans, it can hardly be very
helpful.

Finally, I assume a very close connection between sexuality and religion. Anthropological and
archeological evidence indicate that these two human phenomena are intimately connected. The work
of my colleague William McCready also suggests
that religious world view and sexual self-definition
are acquired in the same process. The challenge of

sexuality forces one to fall back on one's basic world view. One responds to sexual challenge inevitably in terms of one's fundamental interpretive scheme of the cosmos. For even the unreligious, sex is religious—not in the sense perhaps of being "churchy" but surely in the sense of raising questions about the ultimate if not the Ultimate. But if sex and religion are intimately linked, it does not follow that the style with which organized religion has traditionally approached human sexuality is either effective or helpful. All too often religion has been ready to provide answers to sexual problems before the questions were asked. More recently, religion has been providing answers to certain peripheral questions, ignoring more fundamental dilemmas. My assumption is that the role of religion should not be to "answer" sexual questions but to provide illumination and direction to human beings caught in the dilemmas and ambiguities created by their sexual natures. "Man," as Clifford Geertz remarked, "is an animal suspended in the webs of meaning he himself has created." Religion must above all else provide meaning for humankind, and its most important function on the subject of human sexuality is to provide meaning for human sex. Ethical questions, questions about meaning, are surely important, but they are not as important as fundamental meaning, and they cannot be answered until the meaning context has been created. This book is concerned almost solely with the religious meaning of sexuality, not with specific ethical or moral issues. Those I am willing to leave to other writers.

I am therefore not concerned here with the canonical questions of divorce and remarriage for Catholics or the sinfulness of extra- or comarital sex. I do not say these are unimportant questions, but they

are not the subject of this book. If I argue in favor of
sustained sexual commitment, I do so not on canonical or ethical grounds (though I do not reject their
importance) but rather on the basis of analysis of the
dynamics of sexual playfulness. And if I invoke religion in this book, I do so not to support a canonical
or ethical position but because religious symbols
will either illumine the dilemmas of sexual playfulness
or they will be useless as religious symbols to contemporary humans. Humans will then either find
religious symbols that do ratify and reinforce their
sexual playfulness or they will stop being playful and
settle for lives and sex relationships that are dull and
routine.

I intend this essay to be a companion to my
earlier *Sexual Intimacy*. As one who has stumbled
more or less by accident into the business of writing
about sex, I have been struck by the special demands
readers place on an author who discusses sex. Quite
simply put, many readers expect you to say everything at once. You may assume nothing, defer nothing
to a later chapter, leave out nothing. Many readers begin to argue with you at the first paragraph. I
think this is because they feel profoundly threatened
by any discussion of sexual intimacy. A book on sex,
particularly if it has a religious perspective, is sort of
an inkblot into which the reader can project his
frustrations, his hatreds, his anger. If one leaves out
in any given chapter any reference to children, one is
opposed to children. If in another chapter one ne-
glects to mention the frailties and inadequacies of
every human relationship, then one is accused of
having a "romantic," "idealistic" view of sexuality.
It does no good to argue that the matter is treated
elsewhere, or that it should be obvious from the

context what one's point is. In a book on sex it would seem that nothing is obvious from the context.

When faced with such demands from his readers, the author has two alternatives. He can attempt to say everything at once, qualify every phrase, footnote every sentence, cross-reference every paragraph. Or he can assume that what he has to say is intended for reasonably mature adults who are capable of listening to a complex and intricate argument, and who are not waiting to trip him up at the end of every paragraph. In this essay I propose to maintain the latter strategy. Sentences must be judged in the context of their paragraphs, paragraphs in the context of the chapters, chapters in the context of the entire book, and this essay in the context of *Sexual Intimacy*. If I am required to repeat everything I said in my first essay in order to reassure the reader of my sanity or my orthodoxy or my realism, then I shall be writing that essay again. If the reader is trying to pick a fight with me, he will be disappointed to find that I will not fight back.

Thus my argument and my assumptions are laid out clearly at the beginning for all to see. I do not apologize either for the argument or the assumptions. They seem to me to be eminently reasonable. They are, however, sufficiently different from most Christian writing on sexuality as to be disconcerting to many. Even more disconcerting will be the fact that a committed celibate Catholic priest could presume to write on sexual playfulness. Those who reject ideas and authors on principle because they are disconcerting would be well advised to read no further.

12

A long time ago, back before the Vatican Council, I was involved in a lengthy discussion with one of the founders of the feminist movement. In 1960 she was surprised to learn that as a Catholic priest I had no problem at all endorsing the goals of feminism (at least in the rhetoric that was stated then). Having seen what the "woman's-place-is-in-the-home" cultural norms did to well-educated college women in their thirties and forties, it was difficult for me not to be in favor of the feminist movement even before Pope John endorsed it. The discussion turned somewhat gingerly to the subject of sex. "The trouble with you traditionalists," said my friend, "is that you think sex must be linked with love. I quite agree with the impressive Christian vision of marriage, but I don't think that sex needs to be limited to marriage. Modern men and women have discovered that sex can be play, and it does not necessarily have to involve love. You can enjoy sex with strangers, casual acquaintances, the person down the street without there being any psychological intimacy involved."

My friend was deeply committed to her own marriage, and while she and her husband would not define themselves exactly as Christians, she was still willing to admit that the Christian ideal of marriage and the Christian concept of the relationship between sex and love were compelling. If sex were linked with love, then, she conceded, the result was almost inevitably something that looked like marriage. But sex didn't have to be linked with love; it could also be play, and play was casual, spontaneous, freewheeling, open-ended.

I responded with what was the more or less approved "Cana line" of the day: Human sexuality was a serious business; sustained personal relationships required depth, maturity, commitment; shallow, superficial sexual encounters were unrewarding and frustrating. Marriage was a serious attempt to build a common life together, of which sexuality would be a part, an important part, but not the only part. Frivolous and casual relationships might have a short-run psychological payoff, but in the long term they would be harmful and counterproductive. My friend neither agreed nor disagreed; she simply continued to insist that sex need not involve love, and that the discovery (or rediscovery) of the playful elements of sex had changed the entire picture of contemporary human sexuality.

A lot has happened since 1960. Hedonism, which existed in those days as the sophisticated version of such sexologists as the Ellises (Havelock and Albert) and in the adolescent variety of the then-emerging *Playboy* Philosophy, has become a popular and widely heralded sexual theory. Wife swapping, group marriages, alternative marriages, open marriages, "comarital" sex are all hailed as part of the sexual revolution and propagated by some with the dedicated missionary fervor of those who believe they are the wave of the future. We may not remember that hedonism is a very old theory. We ignore the bizarre argument of some of the neohedonists that spouse swapping or group sex reinforces the bonds of middle-class marriage. We rarely observe that many of the advocates of hedonism are dreadfully serious, unattractive people. We never mind that much of the new hedonism is an exercise in chauvinism, with males striving to act out their adolescent fantasies by pressuring their wives into experiments (See Gilbert Bartell, *Group Sex*, New York: New American Library, 1971). And we never notice that the neohedonists represent what is certainly a very small segment of the population. The critical point is that they have taken the initiative in proclaiming the importance of variety and play in sexual relationships. However, we concede too much when we allow them to propound that variety and play in sexual relationships should be sought with a number of different people.

My response to my feminist friend in 1960 was an example of that excessive concession. At no point in the discussion did I deny that casual, transient, "spontaneous" relationships could provide playfulness and variety. I accepted as a given the dichotomy between the serious business of marriage and sexual playfulness. I assumed that playfulness was shallow and superficial. In the face of such argumentation the hedonists will surely sweep the field of battle because it has already been yielded to them.

A couple of months ago I encountered a "with-it" marriage counselor (of vague Catholic antecedents) who repeated the argument I heard from the protofeminist back in 1960. This time I was ready.

"Do your children [both of them under ten] like to play?" I asked.

"Well of course they do."

"And do they play with strangers, casual acquaintances, people they don't care about?"

"That's different," she said, somewhat lamely.

The trouble with "sex-as-play" philosophy, as articulated in its adolescent statement in *Playboy* and now *Playgirl* or in the much more sophisticated version of so-called "scientific" experts, is not that it misunderstands sex. The trouble is that it misunderstands play. Sex is a game, all right, and an uproariously funny one at that; but the "play" crowd has long since forgotten what a game is.

Sex either is playful or it becomes a difficult burden, an obligation, a tension release that produces only minimal satisfaction. A marriage is either a playful relationship, a relationship between playmates (understood here as "mates who play"), or it is an intolerable version. The tango in *Last Tango in Paris* was a dance of death. It was a caricature of the playmate relationship of the *Playboy* Philosophy. It represented, sometimes crudely and tastelessly, the loneliness and despair that lie just beneath the surface of shallow, selfish hedonism. The merit of the picture—and it was not, in my judgment, much of an artistic success—was that it portrayed the loneliness and despair of a sexual relationship without depth, without commitment. The tango was anything but playful.

But neither are many marriages. Depth they may have—particularly when there are children involved—and passion they may generate, but lightness, merriment, playfulness are too often absent.

Watch closely, for example, the electricity between
the husband and wife when they move from one
modality to another. They enter a cocktail or dinner
party. There had been a frantic rush at the end of the
day to take care of the children, dress for the party,
get into the car to arrive no more than a half hour
late. Tensions, conflicts, desires, passions, frustrations build up in the frantic rush to get out of the
house and to the party. When they enter the room it
is almost as though they have interrupted a conversation and must now put on hastily a new set of
masks. There may have been no argument, no overt
conflict, no serious discussion even during the prepa-
rations and trip to the party. Still there was a powerful electricity between them as they came through
the door, and on that electrical current there were
many messages: love, affection, frustration, anger,
hatred, desire, resentment, conflict, weariness, hope.
The current is powerful and cannot be disconnected.
They cannot live with each other in an easy, casual
fashion, yet they surely cannot live without each
other either. (Although as the children grow up, the
marriage will likely go through a severe crisis and
may even end.)

Or imagine the husband and wife stepping into
a hotel elevator in the morning. In the tense silence
between them, the electrical current alternates back
and forth with great intensity. When they are home
there is rarely time for interaction in the morning;
they must get the kids and themselves off to their
respective tasks. But in the unfamiliar, cramped quarters of the hotel room and with the prospect of
breakfast, indeed a whole day, together, the ordinary
context of their relationship is temporarily shattered.
Desire may be heightened but also frustration, resentment, and discontent. It is as though the lines

were overloaded; there is so much being exchanged silently between the two of them. Now in the presence of the embarrassed third party there is silence, tension, and resentment charging the air.

Intimacy in marriage can be oppressively close. It can take on the inevitability of a soggy, humid summer day or a bitter winter's snowstorm. One is simply caught up in it; you cannot enjoy it, you cannot escape from it. The relationship is intricate, complex, subtle, powerful, demanding, and occasionally rewarding, of course. What is missing is a characteristic that might not eliminate any of the messages passing from one to the other but might well transform the significance of those messages. That element is play. One encounters marital playfulness occasionally, and the difference between married playmates and other couples is so striking that one apprehends it immediately. When a husband and wife come into the cocktail party they seem to be laughing with and at each other. Their jests, some of them secret and almost embarrassingly private, bounce back and forth throughout the evening. They enjoy being at the party together, and whatever other messages are on the electrical charges, the message of mutual enjoyment is paramount. They may fight like cats and dogs, but they seem to enjoy that too.

When you intrude into their privacy by being on the elevator with them in the morning, you cannot miss the fact that behind their silence is a teasing, laughing amusement. The strange, unfamiliar confines of the hotel room for such a couple are not an oppression but an opportunity; and the electricity leaping back and forth between them suggests that they are not merely husband and wife, they are playmates.

But what is play and how do we become playful?

That we have to ask this question is evidence that we have forgotten what it was like. The child does not need a definition of play, and no one has to teach him how to be playful. Play is a world unto itself, a game with its own rules, its own parameters, its own constraints. It is real, indeed, terribly real; but it is quite distinct from the mundane world of everyday events. The child does not confuse his game with the rest of life. The boundary lines are firm, but within those boundaries the rules of the game replace the rules of the real world. His game is competitive, imaginative, festive, fantastic; it is intricate, subtle, involved. It is played only with friends, with those he trusts, with those he cares about. Strangers are not welcomed into the game—not until they stop being strangers. The game is spontaneous, but it is also disciplined. Any spontaneity that breaks the rules of the game will destroy it. The game is fun, but it is also serious; it is competitive, but the rules must be strictly observed.

Children can play because they have the fundamental capacity to create worlds of fantasy and festivity that are "real" but distinct from the other real world. From the perspective of the world whose reality is mundane, the world of play is imaginative and perhaps even "unreal." But from the perspective of someone playing the game, the imaginative world is not unreal at all; it just has a different kind of reality.

The tragedy of growing up, for most of us at any rate, is that we lose this imaginative capacity to create a world of play. Even our games are not festive and fantastic but are invaded by the dreadful mundaneness of the ordinary world. Compare nine-year-olds playing baseball (at least the game removed from that awful creation of the adult world,

Little League) with their fathers' golf game. Both age groups play to win, but there is a lightness and a frolic in the game of the nine-year-olds that their fathers rarely match. Winning is important in the game, but when it is over it is no longer important. For his father, on the other hand, competitiveness frequently becomes a way of "proving" his masculinity; winning is a deadly serious business. Unlike the child the adult is incapable of excluding the mundane from the playful.

In the ideal maturation process exactly the opposite should occur. Adults ought to permit the festivity and fantasy of play to carry over and transform their mundane lives. In other words, maturity means becoming more than children rather than less. The playful adult is the person who has kept alive his childhood capacity for dreams and celebration, and has developed the skills required to permit those dreams and celebrations to give shape and color and tone to the totality of his life. For such an adult sex is one of the greatest of games, and the festivity and fantasy, the imagination and resourcefulness that mark the game played in the bedroom with one's spouse simply cannot be contained there. It should permeate the rest of the relationship and the rest of life. Imaginative, challenging, vigorous foreplay precedes sex; but sex in itself becomes foreplay for the rest of life.

Play, of course, is relational. Children may occasionally play by themselves, and they certainly spin elaborate game fantasies without the help of other children. But these fantasies usually involve other people even if they are only make-believe. The child playing by himself rapidly tires of the game and seeks out a friend to invite into his dream world. For a child, playful relationships are relatively easy to create, because neither he nor his friend requires much depth to be able to sustain a game. But adult playful relationships are devilishly difficult to create and sustain. A child need not risk much of himself by inviting another child into his fantasies, his dreams, his celebrations, his festivities. But an adult exposes himself quite completely when he invites another to share fantasy and celebration with him. "Serious," businesslike, responsible relationships come relatively easily; playful ones are difficult if not impossible for most adults. Sex, then, must necessarily be serious, businesslike, responsible. It cannot really be a game, and even casual, transient sex quickly becomes serious despite its superficiality—indeed, probably because of it. One must absolutely and imperatively enjoy casual sex, for if it isn't fun it isn't anything, and the whole thing will be totally devoid of meaning.

It is precisely on the subject of meaning that religion inevitably intervenes in the search for sexual playfulness. The child does not doubt that playfulness is possible. Nor does he doubt that it has a point; he does not need religious symbols to give him the courage to break out of the mundane world into the world of fantasy. While he draws a sharp line between the mundane and the fantastic, it is not one that gives superiority to one world or the other. But the adult, caught up as he is in the cares, the responsibilities, the weariness, the routine of daily life, is not at all sure that it is safe to "pretend," or to admit that that "let's-pretend" world might also be real. The child goes off to the land of Oz with almost reckless ease even though it doesn't really exist. And when he finally succumbs to disbelief in that magical land, the possibility of play is gone from his life. It is, as we shall see in this essay, not easy to develop a sustained playful relationship with one's sexual partner. One can go through the mechanics of foreplay, lasting somewhere between fifteen minutes and one half hour for the typical American couple (according to a study limited, alas, to young college graduates), without the interlude's being anything more than a perfunctory physiological routine. There are obviously some organs of the opposite sex that almost demand that we play with them, and once we do play with them, delightful reactions occur both in our partner and in ourselves. To engage in such activity with a modicum of efficiency is not all that difficult, though a surprisingly large number of married couples are not even capable of advancing that far. To turn the foreplay interlude—that most critical of transitions between ordinary life and orgasm—into an exercise of relaxed, confident, creative, spontaneous mutual fantasy and celebration requires all kinds of skills and sensitivities that seem to be in short supply in the population. And to create a context for sexual relationship for which the foreplay transition is both a symbol and a continuation and a reinforcement takes practice, discipline, patience, perseverance. Many would prefer not to commit themselves.

In other words, foreplay becomes play—as a child understands the word—only in the context of a relationship that is already characterized by qualities of adult playfulness that are hard to acquire, and that many people feel are foolish and unnecessary.

Sex cannot be playful if one does not believe in the possibility of play in one's life, and many of us do not believe in that possibility. In response to the original publication of my previous essay, *Sexual Intimacy*, I received many angry letters from people (mostly women) whose lives were blighted by suffering and sorrow, some of it clearly of their own making. In a grim world of sickness, noisy children, miscarriages, drunken husbands, employment worries, frustrations, disillusionments, and disappointments, can one seriously believe that play is possible, desirable, or necessary? Sex is an obligation, a routine, an interlude. To demand of people who have suffered through and from sex that it be a game is irrational and unjust. One cannot demand anything of anyone in these matters, but if the question is whether play is possible and whether sex can be playful, there is, I think, a very clear answer in the Christian symbol system: Play is indeed possible and is in fact the only adequate response to the Christian message of joy preached in the gospel.

If play is possible for adults and if enjoyment of fun and games is an appropriate response to the Good News we have heard, then sex should become fun and games. Our relationship with our sexual partner ought not to be one of tolerance or obligation or long-suffering acceptance but rather one of sport, delight, and playfulness. To those who say it is no longer possible for them, one must express sympathy—and perhaps a bit of skepticism. Of course they are best able to judge their own cases, but still it must be said that playful sex is not only a legitimate ideal for Christians, it is also an especially appropriate response to the illumination radiated by the Christian symbol system.

In a somber, dull, stodgy, humorless world it might be wrong for sex to be playful, but in a world of joy, confidence, and eager expectation there is no reason for sex not to be playful, and many reasons for it to become an exercise in joy, festivity, celebration, and fantasy. To put the matter somewhat differently, when two sexual partners are firmly committed to each other and seek to become playmates, their efforts are ratified and reinforced by the Christian symbol system, which tells them that such playful joy is an appropriate response to the wheeling, dealing, playful Holy Spirit. When a couple decides— and it is usually an implicit decision—that their sexual relationship should be restrained, constrained, routine, and carefully controlled, they cannot justify it in terms of a religious symbol system. Christian lovers dance and play together because they believe that life, for all its tragedy, is still ultimately a comedy, indeed, a comic, playful dance with a passionately loving God.

It all depends on what meaning we wish to impart to a phenomenon. Clifford Geertz poses the question of what the wink of an eye means. It is, after all, only a physiological reflex—a nervous quirk, a response to a bright light—but it also might be a laugh, a suggestion, a subtle message. But what is the message? Does it mean, "Don't believe me," or "Laugh with me," or "I would like to sleep with you," or "That person is crazy, isn't he?" The physiological movement of nerves and muscles is the same, but what that reaction means to the one who emits it and the one who perceives it depends entirely on their shared interpretation of an eyelid twitch. One can, as Geertz points out, put almost any meaning into it from the most shallow to the most profound.

If such be the case with a blink of an eye, how much more is it true of sexual intercourse! Two people come together in a context in which they have temporarily shut themselves off from the rest of the world. They remove their clothes, they enjoy looking at each other's body, they caress and manipulate one another, becoming increasingly more vigorous and direct in their mutual stimulation. The bodies join, they twist and turn, there are spasms, convulsions, and then relaxation—five minutes, fifteen minutes, forty-five minutes and it is over. But what does the event mean? Is it an obligation? An economic exchange (either in a house of prostitution or in a suburban home)? Is it an interlude that one or both partners experience with loathing and disgust? Is it a routine and absentminded episode? Is it a burst of spontaneous passion? Is it a brief encounter between two people who will never see each other again? Is it part of a great game between two people who have become specialists in playing with one another? Is it a celebration of a relationship that, for all its difficulties and problems, is basically characterized by joyous love? Is it a response not only to the attractiveness of the other's body and person but also to a basically benign and attractive cosmos? Is it an act of play celebrated in the midst of a universe that both lovers believe to be benign and gracious or in an oppressive and absurd universe that can punish and destroy? Have these two lovers created for themselves a world of mutual fantasy and festivity, a world in which they are able to be always a surprise and delight to one another? Or are they grim, determined, serious people desperately seeking that kind of orgasm that they have read in the sex manuals is a proof of their success in lovemaking as a man and a woman? Or are they two angry, hateful, punitive people, who are taking out their vindictiveness toward the cosmos and the rest of the human race by tormenting one another?

The list of questions could be endless. Whether the encounter of man and woman is a playful response to a playful universe or not depends ultimately on whether they believe in the possibility of play, hope, and joy. They can interpret their sexual encounters in almost any way they want; how they interpret them will have a profound influence on both the quality of each encounter and their entire relationship with each other.

There are two reasons why sexual play cannot be something casual and "spontaneous." First, as even fifteen minutes of observation of children at play would indicate, play by its very nature is not casual. It may not be serious as it is in the mundane world, but within its own context the game has norms of seriousness that are indispensable. Doing whatever one wants, or doing what comes naturally, or "letting it all hang out" destroys the game.

Secondly, whether sex is playful or not depends ultimately on what meaning we give to our sexual encounter. Questions of meaning in human life are never easy, simple, casual ones. We can interpret our sex as playful, and within the context of that interpretation we can expend the energies required to see that it becomes and remains playful. But before we can make this interpretation we have to resolve questions about ourselves, about the other, about the human race, and about the cosmos. These issues are anything but casual or trivial.

Paradoxically, play must be very serious, but it will be destroyed by seriousness. As G. K. Chesterton put it, "The more serious the situation, the more playful the Christian must be." One watches an accomplished entertainer like Ann-Margret (and one can like her or not—I confess to finding her resistible) and has to admit that here is an extraordinarily vivid, dynamic, and spectacular entertainer. She gyrates, cavorts, and bellows around the stage and through the audience with an ease, a confidence, an apparent spontaneity that is characteristic of the true professional. Ann-Margret is an absolute expert at playing with an audience. Yet one can tell without even reading her publicity that an immense amount of serious preparation, practice, and discipline went into her act, and that she must be deadly serious about her profession. Each TV special can make or break the career of any performer, particularly that of any whose act depends on torch singing and grinding dance. It is precisely because the special is so serious and she is so serious about her career that her performance must give the appearance of being relaxed, casual, spontaneous. Only discipline, practice, and self-control can enable one to be playful in deadly serious situations. The amateur falls apart and becomes serious in serious moments; the professional becomes brilliantly relaxed, self-possessed, creative. If our sex is to be playful we must become professional.

Most marriages are both too serious to be playful and not serious enough. They are too serious because the burdens, the responsibilities, the discouragements, the frustrations of life make the relationship so heavy, so oppressive, that there is no room for fantasy and celebration. And they are not serious enough because neither partner has expended the effort, the energy, and the discipline or the perseverence, the patience, to become professional in the skills that this particular relationship requires. Hedonism quite properly indicts the oppressive seriousness, but it does not even begin to understand the reasons why a serious commitment to growth of a relationship is indispensable for the play that hedonism superficially exalts.

The blink of the eye is subject to an infinite variety of interpretations, but more complex human activities are less malleable. There is a wide variety of possible interpretations for sexual encounter, but most of them are either gracious or malign. The overwhelming pleasure of orgasm and the fierce physical self-revelation involved are either the hint of something much better or the ultimate absurdity of a punitive universe. If the former is the case, then play is possible. It is the rare husband and wife who do not experience at least the intuition that much more is possible in lovemaking and in the totality of life together and, indeed, in the totality of life itself. When two bodies are pressed together, the flesh soft and smooth, the organs firm and demanding, the passion wild to the point of fury, the rhythms of union building to a crescendo, they are, however temporarily, translated out of the mundane world into one where playfulness seems not only possible but imperative. As they hold each other tight and close, they experience—however fleetingly and however rarely—the hint of an explanation, an explanation of themselves, their sexuality, their love, their life, and of the universe.

The critical question is whether that hint ought to be taken seriously or brushed aside when they return, all too quickly, to the ordinary, mundane world. On some occasions when they are making love to one another they find themselves carried away into a celebration. Ought one to take seriously the possibility that there is a great deal to celebrate?

13

There are a number of painful dilemmas built into the structure of contemporary marital sexuality. On the one hand there is a tremendous biological urge for sexual union reinforced by the psychological theory that says such union is good and healthy. On the other hand there are the friction, conflict, tension, and strain that necessarily build up between two human beings who are forced to live together in close and intimate personal relations. Sexual yearnings draw a man and woman together; interpersonal strains force them apart.

At a deeper level there is the conviction that interpersonal relationships, in particular marriage, are the major source of life satisfaction available to human beings in the contemporary world. A tremendous amount of emotional resources are necessarily involved in seeking marital satisfaction, but so much time and effort must be expended on the difficulties of building a life together that there seems little left over for enjoying the results of a common life. Self-fulfillment is the goal of marriage, but the work necessary to hold the marriage together seems to preclude the possibility of much fulfillment.

There is, then, the serious business of marriage, that of building a life together; and then there is the excitement, the adventure of sexual exploration and play. The two do not seem to fit together very well. Indeed it almost seems as though one must choose, and eventually, for most people, the choice is the common life rather than playfulness. Sexual adventure outside the common life is a solution for very few; it is time-consuming and inconvenient and quickly becomes psychologically painful.

The choices seem clear enough. One either builds a common life without romance or pursues romance without the common life. For the young, the latter alternative seems more attractive; for the older—particularly after the trauma of a divorce—the former seems to be less painful, less traumatic. The risky compromise in between, in which common life characterizes one relationship and playfulness another, is so frustrating in the long run when one relationship or the other either goes sour or they impinge on one another to such a degree that both relationships become intolerable. One cannot have playful, adventurous, exciting, festive, fantastic sex with one person and at the same time build a strong, stable, supportive family life with another.

But how can the conflicts, the tensions, the responsibilities, the burdens, the financial and administrative difficulties, constant problems with the children—all those things that constitute the warp and woof of family living—coexist with playfulness? At the end of a human life, or on anniversary days, one looks back on the struggles and strains, the successes and failures, the defeats and the accomplishments of a common life and realizes that these are what human existence is all about. One may have had to give up some of one's dreams and ideals, but the sacrifice seems worth the effort. Life is a serious business, after all. One may have youthful adventures and perhaps one or two more in mature adulthood, but these are of a different and substantially lesser order of being than is the common life one has built with one's spouse and children.

Or at least so it seems.

The hedonists argue that such a life of bourgeois respectability is dull, weary, and dead. Human beings, they insist, are playful creatures by nature, and they repress the festive, the fantastic, the creative genius, the imaginative, fun-loving, pleasure-seeking elements of their lives at the risk of becoming substantially less than human. The drab, unexciting, unmysterious, unadventurous suburban middle-class marriage may be an efficient economic and social unit, the hedonists tell us; it may be well suited for the production and consumption of wealth and the education of children, but it necessarily represses much of the human personality and stagnates human development and growth. Culture, art, religion, poetry, mysticism, we are informed, all require that humans be able to break away, at least intermittently, from the mundane, the routine, the ordinary, and the commonplace. The stodgy, mediocre American family life, they insist, is a caricature of human sexuality. The furtive, episodic, and unfulfilling release of sexual tension characteristic of such marriages is in its own way even more obscene than sexual promiscuity. Sex without play, without delight, without festivity is, they say, the ultimate in sexual immorality.

The hedonists have a point, though, like all heretics, they confuse part of the truth with the whole of it. Forced to choose between playfulness and somberness, authentic Christianity must choose the former, for a Christian believes (along with Plato) that man is a plaything of God; creation was an act of sport, of playfulness, of creative fantasy and imagination. The Book of Wisdom presents the divine Logos playfully cooperating in God's frolicsome creation of the world. Or, as one of the old Latin versions translates the Greek, *"Jucundabar ante faciem aeius in omni tempore, cum laetaretur orbe perfecto."* ("I was playful before his face all the time when he was rejoicing over the completing of the earth.")

St. Gregory of Nazianzen put the same thought into one of his poems:

For the Logos on high plays
Stirring the whole cosmos back and forth as
He wills into being shapes of every kind.

A contemporary Scripture scholar, Cornelius a Lapide, notes of the Logos that, "In the dewy freshness and the springtime beauty of his eternal youth, he eternally enacts a game before his Father."

Hugo Rahner, in his book *Man at Play* (Herder and Herder, 1967, from which I have lifted the previous quotations), argues that only when we understand the notion of a *Deus ludens* (a playing God) can we understand the notion of *Homo ludens*. Life is joy and sorrow, comedy and tragedy, defeat and victory. Existence is joyful because it is secure in God; it is tragic because it is free, and from freedom come risk and peril. Man, says Father Rahner, "is really always two men in one. He is a man with an easy gaiety of spirit, one might almost say a man of spiritual elegance, a man who feels himself to be living in invincible security; but he is also a man of tragedy, a man of laughter and tears, a man indeed of gentle irony, for he sees through the tragically ridiculous mask of the game of life and has taken the measure of the cramping boundaries of our earthly existence."

Our play, then, is both a celebration of our confidence and an ironic recognition of the fragility of our existence. Rahner quotes with approval the eloquent words of Plotinus: "After all, things at play, play only because of their urge to attain to the vision of God, whether they are the seriousness of the grown man or the play of a child."

Rahner also sees antipation of the Christian vision of *Deus ludens* and *Homo ludens* in the choral ode in *The Frogs*:

> Let me never cease throughout the day to play,
>   to dance, to sing.
> Let me utter many a quip.
> Let me also say much meant in earnest
> And if my playing and mockery be worthy of thy feast
> Let me be crowned with the garland of victory.

The Christian cannot help but agree with the hedonist critique of a life that is mundane and dull. When humans become so rooted in the problems, the cares, the responsibilities of daily life that they cannot break away for festivity and fantasy, they have cut themselves off from the tragic and comic dimensions of human existence. As Robert Neale says in his book *In Praise of Play*, "He who cannot play, cannot pray. He who cannot escape from the responsibilities of work simply will not have time to lift up his head and confront the cosmos and its creator" (Harper & Row, 1969).

This volume is not intended to be a defense of the theology of play. Nor is it an argument justifying the playful dimensions of the human personality and the playful aspects of human existence. I intend to assume that play is justified and indeed indispensable for humankind. I intend to assume that the hedonistic critique of unplayful sex is valid. I take it as axiomatic that a sexual relationship from which all imagination and celebration have been removed is not a Christian relationship. It may very well be an admirable, praiseworthy, responsible, sensible way to live; the religion that underpins it—Stoicism—has always been impressive, but it is not Christianity. Stoic sexuality—puritanism—is not Christian sexuality no matter how much it may claim to be.

But if Christianity agrees with hedonism and its criticism of the unplayful life, it must side with the Stoics in their criticism of the shallow, superficial, rootless life of the hedonist. When the Stoic says romance is not possible if a common life is to be built, the Christian enthusiastically endorses the hedonist's position that life without romance is hardly life at all. But when the hedonist then contends that romance is to be sought outside the common life, the Christian must also dissent. As I argue in this essay, romance apart from the common life cannot survive for very long.

The common life is an absolutely indispensable context for playfulness. Playfulness in its turn is absolutely indispensable to keep the common life from becoming intolerably oppressive. There is surely strain between playfulness and the common life; strain is part of the human condition, that admixture of comedy and tragedy, joy and sorrow, life and death. But one does not solve the problem of strain between two polarities by repressing one or the other part. One can balance a common life and playfulness only when one has powerful convictions that such a balance is possible. And the Christian, being possessed of religious symbols that generate such convictions, ought to be equipped for the struggle to balance the mundane, the ordinary and the fantastic, the commonplace and the playful, the routine and the imaginative. Most of those who profess to be Christian may be unaware of the fact, but it is in that balancing act that one finds the essence of Christian life and, necessarily, the essence of Christian sexuality. Christians are not, of course, the only ones who have grasped this insight. Father Rahner's quotations of some of the Greeks make it clear that others have seen it too. All that can be said is that the Christian vision of a *Deus ludens*, a playful God, gives them an extremely powerful religious symbol to reinforce their search for a mixture of responsibility and playfulness, seriousness and frolic. We may continue to be dull, but to the extent that we are dull we are false to the belief we profess.

Two convictions are necessary: (1) Sex has a built-in strain toward playfulness, which can be resisted only at the price of reducing the payoffs and the binding power of sexual intimacy. (2) Playfulness cannot survive unless it is rooted in the context of a long-term, sustained, total human relationship, one underpinned by the fundamental conviction of the possibility of hope and of love.

The strain toward playfulness in sexuality ought to be self-evident. Indeed most of those who contend that there is little room in life for sexual playfulness do so not on the grounds that sex is inherently unplayful but rather that the other obligations and responsibilities of life make it necessary to limit and restrain sex's playful propensities. If a man and woman would spend as much time playing with one another as their sexual instincts impel them, nothing else would be done.

Most sexual partners are well aware that they impose severe restraints on their sexual exchanges. Remote preparation, foreplay, lovemaking itself are all restrained compared to what they might be. Such restraints are explained on the grounds of no time or energy, other commitments, or even concern for the sensitivities of the other partner. Honesty might lead them to add that fear, uncertainty, shame, and punitiveness are additional motivations for the limitations of their sexual playfulness.

All human events are necessarily limited and constrained. I am not arguing here for the abandonment of restraints. I merely point out that sexual partners know that they could easily be far more playful in their interchanges than they are in fact. At the end of an episode that has been at best undistinguished both the man and woman know that if they had been a little more sensitive, a little more patient, a little more considerate, a little more demanding, a little more challenging, a little more imaginative, the payoff would have been much greater. The man may well think to himself, in effect, "If I had been more affectionate when I came home, more tender through the supper hour, more cheerful during the evening, more fervent, less restrained and inhibited during the intercourse itself, the results would have been more satisfying for the two of us." If she had been more seductive, warmer, more enticing, more insistent on her own pleasure, more aggressive, more unrestrained in her reactions, both of them would have had less guilt about the relative failure of the sexual interlude. It would have been relatively easy to make much more of the episode, but they were both distracted, preoccupied, perhaps resentful and frustrated. What might have been a great event was only a mediocre one.

Even on those occasions when the sexual encounter is uninhibited, unrestrained, and genuinely ecstatic, the man and woman are still aware—and perhaps more poignantly so—not merely that they could much more frequently experience such mutual pleasure but also that it is relatively easy to go beyond where they were even when the satisfaction was great indeed. There are so many things one can do psychologically and physically; there are so many ways that sex can be enjoyed; there are so many ways one can turn on one's partner and be turned on by that partner. The point is that not all sex must be perfect; despite the left-wing puritans, in our limited and imperfect human condition that will never be the case. But most men and women know that they are capable of much more in their sexual lives than they permit themselves to experience and that there is immense room for growth and development in sexual pleasure and playfulness if they can find the time, the energy, and the courage and honesty to seek such development.

There are, of course, some people for whom this awareness of the possibility of development does not seem to exist. Their sexual lives have become so narrow, so cramped, so furtive, so inhibited, so anxious that they take their pleasure with haste, embarrassment, guilt, quickly walling off the experience from the rest of their lives. The feel of finger on flesh for them does not indicate new possibilities for their development but new and unacceptable feelings to be quickly denied.

Sex, then, can be playful; indeed for most peopole it can be more playful than it is. That part of the argument is not difficult to make. But the other aspect of sex, the one that concerns us throughout most of this book, is that playfulness requires permanence, or at least a sustained commitment.

The decisive issue in arguing with the hedonists is whether playfulness is something natural, spontaneous, casual; or, put differently, whether playfulness in its apparent spontaneity is something that comes easily and effortlessly or whether it is rather a skill acquired only by patience, practice, and commitment. The professional "player," the basketball star, figure skater, the chess champion, TV comedian, Las Vegas nightclub singer and dancer, all give the impression of ease and spontaneity; but we know that they are able to appear relaxed, casual, and spontaneous about what they do because they have sharpened their skills and disciplined their responses through long, rigorous, patient practice. The professional basketball guard spots an opening and dribbles through it to the basket with no conscious reflection not because such behavior is "natural" but because long years of effort and practice have so disciplined him that he is able to spot such situations and respond to them with a quickness that is so unreflective that it seems natural, spontaneous, and instinctive. Similarly a professional quarterback comes to the line of scrimmage, glances over the opposition's defense, and changes his play, calling an audible signal to take advantage of a weakness he sees in a defensive alignment. Afterwards he would be hard put to say exactly what his line of reasoning was. That he can size up and react to such a situation is not a sign that he is doing something natural or instinctive or spontaneous but that he is a disciplined, practiced professional.

Skill at any kind of game, then, requires patience, practice, perseverance, commitment. Such characteristics are especially needed when the game requires a partner. The pro quarterback and a wide receiver must play together for a couple of years before they are so sensitive to one another's moves, skills, attitudes, instincts that they fit together like a perfectly balanced, delicate mechanism. A good wide receiver, dashing down the field and noting the sudden switch in the defensive situation, *knows* what his quarterback is likely to do in reaction. Without pausing a moment to reflect or changing the speed of his run he adjusts to what he expects his passer to do. Similarly the quarterback can feel and sense how the receiver will react to the situation. It may be a broken play, but still the ball will be right there on target just as the receiver arrives in place to catch it.

A doubles tennis team, a figure-skating duo, accomplished bridge partners, astronauts on a mission, a jazz combo, a symphony conductor and a soloist (for Chicago it is Georg Solti and Vladimir Ashkenazy)—all these teams are held together by subtle, complex, sophisticated relationships in which cues and signals are given and exchanged so quickly, so adroitly, so unself-consciously that even those who are communicating with each other would be hard put to say how the communication took place. But they have acquired their skills of exchange, cooperation, mutual sensitivity, adjusting one response to another only through a long period of hard, patient, persistent practice.

Just imagine two figure skaters trying to leap about on the ice without ever having practiced together. The audience would surely see at least one serious accident before the night is over.

It is also necessary that there be at least some kind of interpersonal trust and affection between the members of such teams. They don't have to be the closest of friends off the playing field. What is necessary is that they like each other and respect each other enough so that the success of their joint venture becomes more important than discharging individual resentments. If a quarterback is angry at a wide receiver who is getting more publicity than he is, the passes are likely to be ever so slightly overthrown—without even the quarterback's intending it. It would be very risky indeed to be a member of an aerial acrobatic team toward whom other members had deep and abiding resentments. Playing together, in other words, requires practice, cooperation, respect, and some modicum of trust and friendship. One must fit one's patterns to the other's, while the other is at the same time adjusting his. This is a complicated, intricate, subtle, challenging, and ultimately rewarding process; and this is what play is all about.

Even play among children requires that the fellow players make adjustments to the rhythms of each other's play—one that most children make easily and effortlessly. The child who refuses to make the adjustments will either pick up his marbles and leave the playground or find himself quietly but firmly excluded from future games. A "spoilsport" is precisely one who is not willing to merge his own abrasive individuality into the team effort.

But note well that individuality is not lost but enhanced through cooperative effort. A good quarterback looks better when he has a good receiver; a good bridge player operates more effectively with a skillful partner; a good tennis player's talent is enhanced by a skillful partner; a good comedian can be made even funnier by an adroit straight man. One may lose some of oneself by commitment to the joint cooperative effort of the game, but one also gains something new. "He who loses his life shall find it."

Good play is both elegant and fun, but the elegance comes from skill and self-discipline (as in a complex water ballet) and not from spontaneous exhibitionism. Fun comes not from doing whatever you want to do but from meshing one's talents and skills in intricate nuance with those of others. When Wayne Gretzky drives the puck by a goalie he has a good deal more fun than when he fails to score, but his ability to succeed so often comes from both his individually honed skills and the practiced discipline of team play.

Play, then, results from practiced ease. Lots of young men grow up with good arms and good eyes and good coordination, but the great quarterbacks are those who can begin with such raw talent and can discipline themselves through years of work, study, and practice in order to "put it all together" in what seems to be a smooth, effortless, unselfconscious rhythm of play. The "natural" athlete cannot become professional and last in the big-time game unless his natural skills are focused, disciplined, practiced. To be good at anything requires commitment, effort, endurance, patience. Anyone who suggests differently simply doesn't understand what life is all about.

The trouble with the hedonists is not that they overestimate the importance of play; it is that they do not understand the dynamics or the phenomenology of play. They think that in a casual, transient relationship, without care or commitment, play can become possible. They believe that the skills, the discipline, the involvement that are required for success in all other games are somehow or other not required for success in the sexual game. The sexual player, according to the hedonist view, is dispensed from the existential obligations that are imposed on those who would play any other kind of game well. One can, they imply, quickly establish a rapport of easy, practiced, subtle communication with another partner that one has just met. One can engage in a complex, intricate sexual dance with someone to whom no commitment has been made and with whom no particular affection is shared. One can, in other words, play the sexual game according to an entirely different set of rules than are required for every other kind of game that humankind knows.

One can, of course, obtain sexual release from virtually any partner. One can experience a certain kind of thrill from conquering a new partner and from engaging in an illicit or forbidden relationship. But such satisfactions are neither very profound nor very durable and are peripheral to the sexual game. One also can find in casual, transient relationships a certain sort of variety (an argument used by the enthusiastic apostles of "swinging"). If "variety" means coupling with another body, and another and another, there can be no real "relationship" other than the old "slam, bang, thank you, ma'am!" type. If "variety" means variation within the lovemaking, then the one- or two-time encounter provides little opportunity for experimentation and innovation. When two people make love for the first time they are both too deeply concerned with the impression they are making on the other and with their own pleasure and satisfaction to venture into the various forms of pleasure giving and taking. The subtle, sophisticated, implicit communication that makes for variety in human relationships simply does not have time to grow in a brief encounter. They meet, they mate, they separate; and not much else occurs. Playfulness and transiency are contradictory to one another. All the rich, elaborate mystery of another human being's body and spirit simply cannot be discovered except in a long-term relationship. Unless one begins to understand the mysteries of another's personhood, then playfulness and the variety that is the fruit of playfulness will not even begin to exist.

We display that which is consistently best in ourselves only in a context where we have some reassurance and security. If one's idea of sex is merely a routine coupling of bodies, then trust, security, and commitment are unnecessary. But if one believes that sexual playfulness involves the sharing of that which is best in both body and spirit, one must inevitably conclude that time, patience, practice, and commitment are as absolutely essential for the sexual game as they are for any other.

You play with those you care about. You let others play with you only if you are reasonably persuaded that they care about you. This is not an option that one may exercise or not; it is part of the fundamental interpersonal dynamics of the human condition. Play without trust, without confidence, without care, without commitment simply will not persist—indeed it will not even begin. Perhaps the reason why so many of the apostles of contemporary hedonism seem so dreadfully dreary when they talk about play is because they are not very playful people and those relationships they extol are anything but playful. Hedonism may provide variety of a sort, but there is no opportunity to develop the practiced, disciplined interactions with another specific human being that are the absolutely indispensable prerequisites for successful play.

One does not have to make this point for any other game. No one in his right mind would expect the football player, the nightclub performer, the figure skater, the chess champion to be good without practice. No one would expect any member of a team to be instanteously skillful at interacting with other members. The need for practice and skills is so obvious in most playful relationships that only a fool would deny it. Nonetheless, both the hedonist and the puritan seem to assume that humans are born with practiced skills in sexuality, skills that can easily and smoothly be invested in any relationship.

Most young people about to begin their lives together simply will not believe it when they are told that they know virtually nothing about what it takes to be a skilled sexual partner. Their world view demands either that they possess total sexual competence at the very beginning of their relationship or that they acquire it almost instantaneously. The thought that it might take years for them to be skillful lovers—at least as many years as it takes a quarterback and a wide receiver to perfect their style with one another—is simply intolerable. After all, what else is there to the sexual game but manipulating a couple of organs and merging two bodies? What else is a playmate besides someone who can give you pleasure and to whom you can bring pleasure? Why should it be all that difficult?

Similarly those who have been together for a long time may be deeply affronted if it is suggested that they may still be sexual amateurs. Such a suggestion is taken as a nasty reflection of their competence as human beings, man or woman. It may well be, of course, that the greatest athletes are the old pros, people in their late thirties and early forties like George Blanda and Sonny Jurgensen. You may have to be thirty-five to have acquired all the skills of a truly great quarterback. And it may not be all that much different for a lover. In fact, loving another human being makes quarterbacking look easy, and a couple committed to each other on a sustained basis should be coming into their prime skills as lovers in their middle years of life. That most people have long since become satisfied, if not complacent, with skills in lovemaking that have not developed at all may be evidence of many things but surely not that loving is easy. The complex psychological and physiological skills required for intimacy and for intimate playfulness must be learned throughout a lifetime. Whenever we think we have learned it all about loving another human being, then we have in fact retired from the game of love.

The requirement of sustained commitment is not imposed from the outside by a prescient deity who spends a good deal of his time devising ways to make the life of humans miserable. It is rather something that flows from the fundamental dynamic of human relationships. If you are satisfied with superficial, shallow, pedestrian sex, then you can take your pleasure wherever you find it and lead the playboy life of noninvolvement. If you want depth, richness, variety, and playfulness in your sexual expressions, there is simply no other way to have it than to acquire a partner and settle down to a long life of exploration, revelation, experimentation and growth, development, mistakes, learning, progress, effort, patience, practice, and perseverance. It is a very difficult affair (pun intended). It is a very high price to pay for playful sex, but there is no other way to acquire the commodity.

Sustained commitment does not automatically guarantee playfulness, of course. On the contrary, in many, many cases a sustained commitment of a sort coexists with dullness and monotony. Commitment does not guarantee playfulness; it is merely the absolutely essential precondition for it. One might wish that it were otherwise, but in fact it is not, and there is nothing much we can do about it.

Those who argue against permanency in the marriage commitment point out that such permanent commitments frequently are nothing more than a context for a life of mediocrity, exploitation, and frustration. I do not wish to debate the point that middle-class marriage in America is frequently frustrating, dull, and exploitive, but it does not follow that more rewarding and challenging relationships can be found in the so-called "new" sexual forms (most of which, incidentally, are very old). What one calls a relationship is considerably less important than whether there is a sustained commitment to the perennial development of the skills required for human love. It is that kind of commitment and that kind of commitment *only* that can guarantee the growth of the knowledge, the understanding, the affection, the skill, the practiced ease, the disciplined resourcefulness, the creative and insightful spontaneity necessary for sexual playfulness. Anything less than that may not be a caricature of marriage but it is surely a form of human sexuality that is less than it might be. It is a shame when humans settle for something less than what might have been, especially when it might have been had with only a little more courage, a little more trust, a bit more willingness to take risks, a little bit more faith.

The obvious implication of the line of reasoning developed in this chapter is that sexual variety is much more likely to be found in the exploration of the depths and the possibilities of one relationship than in flitting from one shallow and transient encounter to another. The psychological validity of such an insight is, I think, unarguable. That many psychologists are reluctant to apply it to sexuality, while readily applying it to other forms of behavior, is evidence that the psychological profession is not always willing to follow its own insights, particularly when they seem to ally them with the traditional wisdom.

For some people, particularly the young, the important point is that playfulness can only be achieved in the context of a sustained commitment. For many others, particularly the not-so-young, the important point is that sexual playfulness can indeed be achieved in a marriage relationship, and that the relationship is never too old to be reborn. It is not necessary to sell the young on the possibility of love or a need for variety within it, but the not-so-young have often made their peace with the absence of variety, think they can do without it, and may even be convinced that it is not possible to achieve. The ultimate conclusion of such existential pessimism is that variety probably is not a good thing after all.

It is precisely at that point that we must turn to our religious symbols. Is variety good? Is variety necessary? Is variety possible? Is there any room for diversity, excitement, novelty in the human condition?

The Christian response to the mystery of variety, plurality, diversity is the symbol of the Holy Spirit, that dimension of the Deity that represents creativity, spontaneity, diversity. If the principle of unity is the Father, the principle of multiplicity and diversity is the Spirit. She is a wheeling, dealing, whirling, twirling, dancing, darting poltergeist Deity, who flits and leaps, spins and dives, dashes in madcap movement through the cosmos, flicking out sparks of creativity and vitality wherever she goes. (In Ireland I think she becomes a leprechaun.) The Spirit is a howling, raging wind, blazing, leaping fire, passionate, protective dove. She blows where she will, stirs up what she wants, speaks to us with the howling of a hurricane or the gentle touch of an evening breeze in the summertime. She calls forth that which is best, most generous, most giving, most risk taking in ourselves. She stirs us up out of complacency, mediocrity, monotony, routine. She is the Spirit of life, of vitality, of excitement, of adventure. She is the Spirit of play, and, together with the creative Word, she dances and sings and claps her hands, as God the Father produces his splendid, variegated, excessive—indeed half-mad—universe. It may even have been the Holy Spirit who poured the cups of the wine of love that intoxicated the creative Father to produce the wild, manic splendor of his creation. The sins against the Holy Spirit are those of despair, giving up, settling down, and not seeking more.

Can one believe in this madcap, merry Spirit and still believe that playfulness is unimportant, unrequired, indeed impossible in human sexuality? One can, perhaps, but then one is not a Christian.

14

Part of the excitement of any game is its mystery. One does not know how the game will end; indeed, one can't be absolutely certain what will happen in the next moment. One may know the "moves" of those one plays with, but yet, for all the knowledge and skill one may have acquired in playing the game, the others are still a source of constant surprise. As the most intimate of games, sex is also the most mysterious. One can live with another human being for years and still not even begin to plumb the mystery of that other person. The more one knows about the other, the more one discovers there is to be known. The very fact that we discover something about the other and bring that particular aspect of his mystery into the open, the more his deeper mysteries begin to actuate themselves in his personality. The more we know them the more strange they become. Another human is either a closed and uninteresting book or a constant and endless source of fascination. Whether he be interesting or not depends as much on our definition of and response to him as on any intrinsic quality of his own nature.

Perhaps the greatest weakness in the preparation that young people receive today for marriage is that no one tells them that life together will be and ought to be an ongoing series of surprises, of discoveries made, of sudden and illuminating bursts of understanding and self-revelation. New puzzles, obscurities, and secrets will be ever present to be probed, explored, and understood. Young people know that there is pleasure and fascination in discovering the body of the other and permitting one's own body to be discovered by the other, but that part of the mystery of revelation and self-discourse is relatively uncomplex. A man may indeed go through decades of married life and understand very little of either the physiology of female sexuality or the physiology of his wife. Still, learning what gives a woman pleasure and what in particular is pleasure to *his* woman is relatively simple compared to the understanding of the deeper mystery of the human personality that creates the context of his wife's sexuality and that is focused so sharply in the ambiance of their sexual encounters. Similarly, the woman may not be particularly interested in discovering what really turns her husband on, but after a while she avoids knowledge on the subject only at considerable effort. The mystery of who and what her man is in the depths of his soul, however, is one about which she can remain serenely unaware throughout the duration of her marriage.

As an absolutely indispensable prerequisite, then, for sexual playfulness, a man and a woman must be determined to get to know one another, which means that they must be determined to commit themselves to endless exploration of the heights and depths and breadths of the mysteries of each other's selfhood. We can only understand another person's sex when we can grasp it in the context of the totality of who and what he is, and that is a lifelong challenge. The more we know the other person, the more influence we have over him. The more we permit the other to know us, the more influence we surrender to him. The greater our knowledge of the other, the more erotic our relationship will become. The process of exploring another's personality is extremely erotic, much more so, in fact, than exploring the other's body, though the two processes go on simultaneously, heightening and reinforcing the pleasurability of both. It is relatively easy, it turns out, to live with a stranger, but we cannot play well with one, no more than can a quarterback and a wide receiver who do not know each other. If one wishes to have playful sex, then one must accept the burden of endless exploration, but one should also understand that after a while the exploration becomes not only a burden and a challenge, but an adventure and reward in itself. To explore the depths of someone else's personality is the most erotic thing a human being can do, and when that exploration is reinforced and facilitated by sexual lovemaking, the lovemaking becomes an episode in a grand adventure, taking on an intensity of pleasure that it would otherwise not have. There are, of course, costs incurred in the acquisition of intimate knowledge and influence over another. The heaviest cost is that one permits the other to have knowledge of and influence over oneself. In addition, time, that most precious commodity in our busy society, is required, as is patience, tact, taste, and courage. It is much, much easier to buy a copy of *Playboy* or advertise in one of the spouse-swapping journals.

From the secure perspective provided only to the celibate outsider, I am always amused by how confident husbands and wives are that they understand their spouse perfectly when it is quite clear, even to the most casual observer, that they understand little if anything about their partner. Somehow or other it is a sign of failure, of inadequacy, of ineptitude to admit that the spouse is a mystery that one is only beginning dimly to understand. In truth, such an admission is a sign of the beginning of wisdom.

After a number of years together there are some things we do know about our spouses: what kind of food they like, what their musical tastes are, what kind of drinks they are likely to order, what kind of mood they are likely to be in in the mornings, how they respond to sickness, inconvenience, stress. This capacity to predict some of their responses lulls us into the complacent conviction that we know everything there is to be known, we understand everything that is to be understood. Of course, the other party may know some things about us, but he is remarkably unperceptive and really doesn't understand us at all; we understand him, though. Oddly enough, he feels exactly the same way.

There is a substantial difference between knowing some things about another human being and *knowing* that other human being. Each one of us is aware of how complex, intricate, and baffling we are even to ourselves. Anyone with even a small capacity for self-examination knows that he is a bundle of mysteries, enigmas, and contradictions, but somehow it is difficult to face making the leap from accepting our own complexities and mystery to realizing that everyone else is as baffling as we are. "My husband is an open book; I am a mystery." "My wife is transparent; I am an enigma." It is a totally unreasonable position, but still a useful one that we are most reluctant to give up.

A young man takes unto himself a wife. He acquires a traveling companion, a housekeeper, a sexual partner, a joint administrator, a potential parent. Her body is delightful to hold, a joy to possess even though he is awkward and uncomfortable in their early attempts at sexual union, and she is neither as responsive nor seductive as her warmth and affection before marriage suggested she would be. Still, they work out some sort of minimal level of sexual adjustment and settle down for their life together. He discovers that she is not quite the person he thought she was when he decided that he should marry her. She can be moody, unpredictable, sometimes very unreasonable. They get along well enough together, and there are satisfactions and rewards as they build a common life and begin to raise their children. They quarrel and fight, make up and love, and slowly develop a long agenda of frustrations and anger and hurt that they cannot or will not discuss. She is a good wife—not quite the kind he had expected but better than most. In any event, he understands her, knows what is necessary to keep her happy and what must be done to reduce the strains and tensions in their joint life to a reasonable minimum. What more, after all, can be expected in this very imperfect world we live in?

And yet he has married a stranger; he lives with a stranger (and she does too). No one ever told him that a spouse was a mystery and that one must devote considerable time and effort to probing the recesses of that mystery. His wife is much like all other women, although in many ways she is quite unique and special. He must value and appreciate her specialness, and he understands her and is able to keep her in line by yielding on the things he must yield on and partly by insisting on the things he knows she will yield. The gene combination that produced her physiology is a combination that never existed before and will never exist again. She comes to marriage with a personality, a value system, and a series of interpretive schemes, a fantasy life, a collection of longings, hungers, fears, anxieties that are totally her own. Her social class, her ethnic group, her religion, the places she grew up in—country, region, neighborhood—the kinds of friends she had, the schools she went to, her adolescent sexual experiences, her relationships with her mother, father, siblings—all of these, combined with the major cultural events of her adolescence and youth and the genetic code of her biological being, produced a complex, delicate, mysterious, fascinating woman who is reduced to a series of propositions and predictions only at the risk of devastating misunderstanding. A husband may be able to sort out and organize some of the more obvious characteristics and behavior, but because he knows how she is likely to respond in given sets of stimuli, it does not follow that he has the foggiest notion of why she so responds—and she may not herself.

She has shared her body with him and a good part of her life space; she has also shared some of her more obvious moods, fears, hopes, and dreams. But there are vast areas of her selfhood that are still intensely private and that she does not want to share or does not know how to share or could not share. It is not necessary for him to know everything about her; there are some things that he need not know, other things he should not know, and still others he will never know. None of this really matters, though. What counts is that if they are to be playmates there is a good deal more that he can and must know. Sometime during the course of their marriage the husband must decide that his wife is an open book, pleasant enough to live with but containing few mysteries and challenges; or he must decide that she is endlessly fascinating and he will devote the rest of his life to her in pleasured fascination. He will encourage her mystery and her uniqueness, because by permitting her to live more fully the mystery she is, he is freeing her to be an enticing, seductive, pliable, playful, aggressive, demanding, yielding lover. And he can stop the pretense of *knowing* her, which is so stilting and limiting to her, him, and their life together.

The decision-point of the husband's making up his mind whether his wife is a mystery or a transparency is of critical importance for their marriage. It is, of course, a decision that can be reversed. He may discover to his chagrin that her mystery and uniqueness do not indeed fascinate him, and he may have to make another decision to go back to the more placid plateau of unquestioning coexistence in order to keep the family together. To retreat from intimacy is tragic, but to deny that it may be necessary or a decision consciously taken is to refuse to admit the complexity and difficulty of interpersonal relationships. "Getting to Know You," as the song from *The King and I* avers, is great fun; still, many husbands and wives think that that period is far behind them in their life together. Perhaps it is, but when the period of getting to know someone is over, the period of playfulness is over too.

Janet and Lawrence had been married fifteen years. All their friends thought it was a happy marriage. They were a handsome couple; they had two cars, a beautiful home, apparently all the money they needed. Their three children were attractive and well behaved. Janet was perhaps a bit too compulsive about her family responsibilities; Lawrence was maybe a little overcommitted to his career as an architect. She might have been better off if she got out of the house more; he might have been better off if he were in it more. Still, compared to most of their friends they seemed to have an ideal marital adjustment.

And then suddenly Janet walked out. She was tired of Lawrence and wanted a life of her own. There was no other man, really, although she was close to having an affair with a divorced friend of theirs. She didn't hate Lawrence and still loved their children, but life with him had become intolerably dull and boring. She wanted to begin to live again.

As the two of them talked, it became clear that they were total strangers. Two years of dating, a year of engagement, and fifteen years of marriage; yet they knew almost nothing about one another. They were strangers who shared the same house, the same children, and sometimes the same bed (though not that very often anymore). But they knew less about each other than Lawrence knew about some of his professional colleagues and Janet did about some of her friends in their town. Their relationship had deteriorated into nonexistence.

Lawrence had always been fiercely competitive in everything he did. On the athletic field, in school, in his work he was driven to excel. He wanted to be the very best, because his father, whom he adored, had been the very best. His competitiveness was not abnormal but it was very strong. He had seen in Janet a warm, witty, charming young woman who would create for him an atmosphere of graciousness and sophistication as respite from the battles of the professional world. Janet had a weak father and an overpowering mother. She had seen in Lawrence a strong, competent male who would free her from the need to worry compulsively about "responsibilities," which her mother had drummed into her. It seemed like a perfect match.

It was and it wasn't. There were aspects of Lawrence's personality—his strength, his drive, his assertiveness—that Janet desperately needed. And there were aspects of her personality—laughter, elegance, intelligence—that he needed. But unfortunately they rarely saw these dimensions of one another. For all his competitiveness, Lawrence was afraid of women (just as his father had been). He didn't know how to be anything but diffident when he encountered resistance or opposition from a woman. Janet's network of compulsive responsibility—she spent weeks working on a Christmas card list each year—was designed to compensate for the guilt she felt over the powerful, passionate drives she had to work so hard to control.

Janet had not the slightest idea that her husband was afraid of women, and especially of her. In fact, when she was told she could not believe it—even though everyone else who knew Lawrence could see his fear after about five minutes. Similarly, Lawrence had no notion of the wild furies of anger, hatred, love, and ambition that stirred in his wife's soul. When he was around she seemed to be dull and pale, though he would quickly add that she was a fine mother and did a great job with the children. Everyone else knew that she was part witch and part bitch—the sexiest woman on the street. But the flare and the fire that she displayed at their dinner parties quickly died when the guests left, and she became the dumpy housewife her husband had always taken for granted.

Their sex life mirrored the rest of their relationship. Janet hated herself for it, but she entered marriage a prude, ashamed of her body and terrified at the thought of intercourse. She was not exactly frigid in bed, but she was almost totally passive. A coquette at cocktail parties, she became shy and embarrassed in the bedroom. Even after a decade and a half of marriage she found it almost impossible to undress in the presence of a man. Her body, supremely graceful when she walked down the street, became awkward and ungainly as soon as it lost the protection of clothes. She assented to intercourse whenever she was asked, but her lack of enthusiasm was obvious.

Lawrence had absorbed from his family environment the belief that the fears and anxieties of a woman should be deferred to always. His wife turned out to be a weak, frightened woman. She wasn't the kind of person he thought he had married, but he was still responsible for her. He would protect her and humor her peculiarities. He "lost interest" in sex because, as he put it, it didn't seem fair that he should be the only one enjoying it. He would not admit it to himself, but he was terrified at the thought of what might happen if he tried to force beyond his wife's compulsiveness and prudery. So he lost himself in his work and the success it brought him. He thought of his family as a successful joint venture in child rearing.

It was a nice arrangement. There were no risks on either side, or so it seemed. Neither party got what they had expected originally in sex or interpersonal support, but the adjustment, while at a low level of payoff, seemed to work. They had mutual interests in art and music, friends, their house, their social life, their children. It was foolish to expect anything more from marriage.

They still had hazy memories of the dreams of each other's strength they had had when they entered marriage, and each still had sexual fantasies. There were times, at night after a party, perhaps, when Lawrence would have a powerful fantasy of ripping the clothes from Janet's body, spending the rest of the night in a wild sexual orgy composed of all manner of unspeakable things. He quickly dismissed such images as adolescent foolishness; still, he would have liked to be able to be an adolescent fool with his wife. Part of his fantasy was that midway through the orgy she would turn on him, take the sexual initiative, and overwhelm him. There was never any danger of something like that happening in the real world.

But Janet's fantasies were remarkably similar— though they did not involve her husband. She was ashamed of it, but the image of a strong, overpowering man ravishing her was frequent and compellingly vivid. Her imagination lingered on every tiny detail of the assault. While the assault was always tender, it was also a violent sexual experience that forced her out of her shame and turned her into a passionate respondent first and then into an aggressor, matching violence with violence. Furthermore, despite her prudery (probably because of it), she had strong exhibitionist fantasies of being stripped and exposed, fantasies that were as delightful as they were terrifying. In both fantasies, of course, her doubts about her own worth and attractiveness as a woman were removed by the forceful actions of others, the kind of actions that were completely absent in her marriage. Unlike Lawrence, she was unable to lose her frustrations in work. Her moving out was an act of desperation.

Janet's and Lawrence's fantasies, then, were as potentially complementary as was everything else about their personalities. Each had chosen the right partner in marriage on solid intuitive if not explicit grounds. But a pattern had developed in their relationship that, instead of playing to each other's strengths, reinforced their weaknesses. They were bringing out in each other exactly the opposite of what both of them needed and suppressing exactly what was needed.

There were psychological reasons for such a vicious circle. Therapy may well be an important part of any rehabilitation of their marriage, but neither Lawrence not Janet was particularly neurotic. Their personality problems certainly helped them in their implicit conspiracy to live together as strangers for fifteen years. but if they are to salvage anything of their life together, they must begin to get to know one another. Fifteen years late is better than never.

Janet was a beautiful, intelligent, complex, challenging woman. To explore the subtleties of her body and spirit would have looked to many men like the opportunity of a lifetime and an opportunity for a lifetime. Her husband didn't see any mystery at all. Lawrence was the kind of vigorous, dynamic, active male that many women find irrestibly fascinating. If he had wanted to be unfaithful it would have been easy. Janet fled him because he was utterly and unbearably dull.

Because they did not know one another they had no influence over one another. Without influence there can be no possibility of growth within a relationship. By "influence" I mean the ability to obtain desired behavior from another human being. The word has taken on bad connotations in our society, but it is impossible for there to be any close human relationship without influence. By the very fact that we love someone he or she has influence over us. And by the very fact that we are loved we have influence over the one who loves us. Influence in intimate relationships can be bad or good; it is good when used to promote the growth of the best dimensions of another's personality and bad when it is used to manipulate and constrain him. We all know how to get something from those who are close to us. We nag or sulk or have a temper tantrum. We know that the other will cave in when we use certain techniques to obtain a desired result. Neither person grows in such an exchange, but in many intimate relationships it is the only use of influence known.

There is another kind of influence that goes far beyond manipulation. It is based on a knowledge of the other person that goes much deeper than knowing what kind of pressure will force him to cave in and do what we want. Such knowledge comes from a serious and sustained exploration of the depths of the other's self. When we have this knowledge we have immense power over the other—to hurt him, indeed, but also to free him. With our knowledge we become skilled at creating an environment in which the other is almost certain to respond the way we want—and the way that the best in him wants.

Janet wanted a lover who would break through her compulsions, fears, guilts, and prudery so that she could give free rein to her wild, creative, passionate personality. She married Lawrence because she sensed—perhaps not in so many words—that he was such a man. It seemed to her that she had made a mistake. In fact she had not. He had the capabilities to be such a husband. If she had gotten to know him she would have discovered his fear of women and also his longings to be the passionate lover she wanted. If she had studied his behavior, his responses, his cues, she would have been able to devise a strategy that would virtually compel him to break through his fears. It would not have been merely a matter of encouraging him but of understanding his fear of women and systematically demolishing that fear.

Similarly, if Lawrence had realized how much his wife wanted to be free of her compulsions and sexual passivity, he would have perceived that a strategy of refusing to tolerate her endless hours of worrying over Christmas card lists might have freed her. Instead of accepting her compulsions he should have simply demanded that they stop. She would have responded quickly and even gratefully. Furthermore, he could have swept aside her prudery and insisted on undressing her himself every night instead of letting her sneak away to the bathroom to change. She might have resisted in terror at first—but not for very long, since the delights from such rough treatment would have been too great.

It was not ill will or neurosis (though there was some of both in their relationship) that kept them from dealing effectively with one another. It was ignorance, an ignorance that was totally unnecessary.

But why do we know so little about those who are close to us? There are three reasons, I think. First, it never occurs to us that we are living in a house with a mystery that can be a source of endless fascination and enjoyment. We think that we know all there is to know of the other and simply stop learning more. After you have been married ten years, what is there left to learn? The answer is that there is an immense amount to learn, but most people simply won't believe it.

Second, we are too busy thinking about ourselves and worrying about what the other is thinking about us to try to figure out what is going on inside him or her. Janet was disgusted with herself, frustrated with her marriage, disappointed with Lawrence, and guilty for having failed him. But in all of these emotions (and in the comparable ones in Lawrence) there is not the slightest hint of curiosity about the fears, the dreams, the expectations, the disappointments, the hopes of the other. If Janet had turned her attention away from her own failures and from Lawrence's inadequacies to wonder about the real Lawrence, she might have discovered his fear of women. In the process she would have taken her mind off herself and might have begun to see the possibility of excitement in their relationship. But Lawrence had long since stopped being a mystery and had become merely part of the scenery, to be accepted unchanged, unchanging, and unchangeable.

Finally, to explore the mystery of another human is work, and we are lazy. It is also risk, because we must reveal ourselves in the process of constraining another to reveal himself. If Lawrence had worked up enough energy to probe into the subtle complexities of his wife's sexual fears and longings, he inevitably would have revealed much about his own sexuality in the process. It would have been a delightful interchange but also dangerous. No telling where things might have gone—though probably not to the divorce court.

But how do we get to know someone else? Let's suppose we acknowledge that we live with strangers. How do we break through the strangeness?

First of all, we pay attention to what we already know but have not bothered to interpret. Lawrence knew—and resented—the kind of men Janet seemed to enjoy. He knew the sort of person she was likely to spar with in her bright, witty chatter. They were men like himself. When Janet was not around he could behave that way with other women. Such exchanges may not be seriously intended but they are of course filled with sexual overtones, invitations, and responses. If Janet liked to flirt with tough, aggressive, demanding men, and if he could be that way, then maybe his gentle diffidence in the face of her passivity was the result of a complete misreading of the situation. He had all the facts; he simply hadn't put them together and interpreted them.

Second, we learn from cues that have been there all along but that we have missed. There are aspects of the mystery of our intimate stranger that are easy to see but we have not noticed. Janet knew that her husband was a hard-driving professional with almost limitless ambition, but around her he was dull and uninteresting. She was torn between thinking that he was undersexed and that she was unattractive. But if she had been at all curious about probing into the mystery that was her husband she would have noticed rather quickly that he tended to be very quiet when meeting a woman for the first time. "Why, Lawrence is shy?" she might exclaim in disbelief. "He's afraid of women?" And it would dawn on her, "Good heavens, he's afraid of *me*!" There are no easy ways out of any human problem, but if Janet had come upon this insight early in their marriage she might have had an exciting and enjoyable time leading this man away from his fears of women while capturing him completely in her femininity. Changing the focus from "What's wrong with him?" and "What's wrong with me?" to "What can I do for him?" might have effected a major transformation in their relationship. The facts were all there; she simply hadn't looked at them.

Finally, we must probe beyond the facts about the intimate stranger to get at the real person. There are times and places when people talk about themselves, sometimes in response to our questions, more likely in response to our interest and affection. Janet knew that Sunday breakfast was one of the few times in the week when Lawrence liked to relax, expand, and talk about himself, his work, his plans. She did her best to cut such sessions short because Sunday was one of those days when her schedule of "ought-to-be-doing" was particularly long. But it was during that half hour on Sunday morning that Lawrence was most open, most vulnerable, most easy to probe and explore. The trouble was that she didn't think there was anything to explore. Instead of guaranteeing privacy for that half hour in which she could snuggle up to him with affection, she would wait impatiently, car keys in hand, for the session to end so that she could get on to the important things.

Janet was most likely to be expansive at the end of the evening over a second drink after the TV news. Since Lawrence had given up using such occasions as a prelude to sex (not that he ever tried very hard), he turned on Johnny Carson and became absorbed in the screen while his wife made seemingly pointless and inane comments about herself. If he had thought there was any mystery at all left in this intimate stranger, he would have turned off the TV, put his arm around his wife, listened very carefully to what she said, and discovered a very different woman from the one he thought he was married to.

It all sounds very calculating. Our current cult of spontaneity has led us to believe that such careful, systematic, even devious exploration of the personality of another is dishonest and even immoral. The loud, aggressive, frequently punitive behavior of the encounter group is supposed to be virtuous, and the persistent, gentle, indirect probing of the intimate stranger is thought to be wrong. Still, all the encounter sessions in the world could not cure what is wrong with the marriage of Janet and Lawrence. An encounter session might reveal to them that they are strangers; it could never make them friends.

What will become of them? I would like to be able to say that their problems were solved, but I cannot. All that I can say is that they have begun to see the problems and are trying, indeed trying very hard. That is all that can be asked of anyone. Janet and Lawrence—like most of us—will have to keep trying for the rest of their lives.

Playfulness may seem to be so heavy a burden, so complex a responsibility, so difficult a task that we might be tempted to give it up and settle for routine mediocrity, which if it is not much fun is not nearly so demanding. Life is hard enough without adding more mystery to it. If one has to work so hard in order to be playful, maybe play isn't worth the effort.

But in fact, probing the mystery of another human being is not preparation for the game, it is the game itself. Getting to know someone is not merely a prelude to eroticism, it is vividly erotic in itself. One gets to know another human being not by serious, sober, dour, and unimaginative cross-examination but by playing with the person. It is in times of fantasy and festivity, merriment and frolic that another person is most likely to reveal himself. Precisely at those times the guards, the defenses, the masks are most likely to be down. We do not force the mysteries and the secrets out of another human being; we seduce them out by attention, affection, encouragement, reassurance, and laughter. To tease slowly the body of

the spouse from indifference to a height of passionate desire is as erotic, if not more so, than the
culmination of the teasing process in orgasm. Or to
put it more precisely, sexual satisfaction that comes
at the end of a slow, gentle, seductive prelude is
infinitely more satisfying than one that is quickly,
hastily, and urgently experienced. An analogous process is at work in probing the mysteries of the other's
personality, in which sexuality is necessarily a critical dimension but not the only one. We explore the
other's personality as we explore her sexuality—slowly,
gently, encouragingly. The technique of seduction
persuades her to share ever more of her endlessly
fascinating selfhood with us. It is work, perhaps, but
it is delightful, enjoyable, and playful work.

Our friends Janet and Lawrence might be ap-
palled at the thought that after fifteen years they
must begin over again almost as perfect strangers.
Worse than that, they must begin as strangers with a
long agenda of frustration and shared antagonisms.
Still, they might look at it differently. Lawrence might
consider that, much to his surprise, he is living with
a mysterious, fascinating stranger, one whom it would
be a great pleasure to get to know. He must begin
again, or begin for the first time, to discover what
her sexual needs, pleasures, and fantasies are. But
while he is learning about her sexually he must at
the same time begin to get to know who she is. This,
too, can be a pleasure so overwhelming that it can
transform his whole life. Furthermore, the fact that
all of this is in some fashion a way of making up for
and reversing past failures can make the experience
even more rewarding.

Janet, for her part, could make the same assumptions and embark upon the same pleasurable
adventure of winning for herself this attractive strang-

er who lives in the same house with her. For both of them, of course, the critical decision is to redefine each other from being an open book to being a fascinating stranger. This is not easy to do at the beginning of a marriage and much less so after many years have passed. But it is still possible, and when the spouse becomes an intimate, mysterious stranger, an enticing, irresistibly attractive stranger, the stage is set for sexual play to begin. The players may begin as amateurs, but so long as they realize that there is much to learn, there is no reason why they should not eventually become professionals.

Those of us who were raised in a rationalist Cartesian world, in which science confidently expected to be able to explain everything, manipulate everything, solve everything, do not like mysteries. They are an affront to our rationality and to our Enlightenment optimism. Religiously a mystery was something that had to be believed under pain of mortal sin, that undigested lump of religious truth for which we could not give a rational defense. We read mystery stories because we expect solutions at the end. A mystery then is either a puzzle to be solved or an obscure doctrine to be swallowed. Scientific philosophers (more frequently than scientists themselves) confidently predicted that soon there would be no mysteries left, and theologians like Rudolf Bultmann said that it is impossible to see mystery in a bolt of electricity across the sky when we can control electricity with a flick of a light switch. When we hear that sex is mysterious, that our sexual partner is a mystery, and that sex cannot be playful unless we recognize its mysteriousness, we are affronted. Sex is, after all, a biological function. Skill can be acquired by learning certain bits of biological information. Sexual hang-ups are the result of either childhood experience or oppressive social structure or old-fashioned religious dogmas. It is an ordinary biological function; how can it possibly be a mystery?

But the younger generation is fascinated by mystery. It realizes that science cannot explain everything, and the best scientists no longer purport to do so. The cosmos is not a machine to be understood and manipulated but a mystery to be explored. Astrology, the I Ching, folklore, occult wisdom are all to be explored, because they might reveal hints and secrets about the meaning of life and about how humans ought to live. As Father Charles Meyer points out in his brilliant book *Man of God* (Doubleday, 1970), we are now moving from the mystagogic to the mystadylic era; that is to say, from a time when we explained mysteries away as puzzles to be solved to a time when we explore mysteries for the secrets to be found there. Sex, like everything else in the world, is indeed ordinary and commonplace; but it shares intimately in the fundamental mysteries of the universe. Why is there anything at all? Why is there a struggle between good and evil? Why is there both unity and diversity? He who thinks that sex is only mystery blinds himself to the ordinariness of human life, but he who thinks that it is only biology blinds himself to the mystery that pervades the cosmos. Mysteries, as any addict to Nero Wolfe, Agatha Christie, Ngaio Marsh, Ross McDonald, and Ellis Peters knows, are fun. And the greatest mystery of all, the mystery of why I am and where I am going, ought to be the greatest fun of all. The passion, power, the pleasure, the pain of sexual intimacy are deeply involved in ways we only dimly perceive with that agonizing question. As we find that other who is our love, we also find ourselves, and in the process the two of us may begin to find the Other who is our Lover.

In the mystagogic world mysteries are sacraments, revelations of great secrets, and not so much obscure puzzles as dazzling rays of light. Sex, then, is mystery, sacrament, revelation. To discover who our lover and ourself really are is to discover something fundamental about the cosmos.

Or as St. Paul says, sexual union is a great sacrament, a great *mysterion*, that reveals the intimacy of God's union with his creatures. We may be content to write off our sex life as a prosaic, pedestrian, biological function. When we do that we miss something the great mystics and the great lovers, the great poets and the great visionaries down through the ages have perceived. When a man and woman are locked in an embrace they come for a few brief seconds close to the core of the greatest Mystery of them all.

15

The *Playboy* centerfold is an erotic picture, crudely, grossly erotic, and appeals primarily to adolescent sexual fantasies. The larger the body organs, the more sexual pleasure is promised. By her smile, her deportment, her casual invitation, the Playmate of the Month promises a fun-filled romp. No hang-ups, no involvements, no commitments, no furniture to buy, no risk of being tied down, no extra responsibilities—just fun and games now, as soon as you want, however you want it, whenever you want it. Images of play are there for the asking; one just has to plunk down a dollar. (If you are a woman, you have now achieved the marvelous equality of being able to plunk down your dollar for a copy of *Playgirl*.)

Let us leave aside the traditional concern over whether the *Playboy* centerfold is a "dirty" picture. (There are images to be found on the walls of the Vatican Museum and the ceiling of the Sistine Cha-

pel that are more erotic.) Whatever the deficiencies
the centerfolds of *Playboy* and *Playgirl* may have as
part of the ancient tradition of erotic art, one must
still observe that the play they promise is phony.
First, the buxom young woman is not in fact prepared to play with anyone. She is posing for a picture for money and the considerable amount of fame
and attention it will bring. She is not prepared to
play with the cameraman taking her picture or the
Playboy buyer who stares at her goggle-eyed. The
invitation in her eyes, her smile, and the arrangement of her body may be an invitation to fantasy, but
it is not in fact anything but an invitation to look.
Looking may be fun, but it's not all that much fun.
The *Playboy* Philosophy, in fact, considers sex to be a
spectator sport where participation is fantasy. The
pro football fan not only admires Jim McMahon's
ability to throw a pass, but he also identifies with
him on the field. In fantasy he leaves his seat in front
of the TV and descends to the gridiron and the battle
being played out there. Similarly, the sexual spectator projects himself into the scene depicted in the
centerfold and becomes involved in the actual game
of sex to which the Playmate of the Month is inviting
him.

A spectator sport may be diverting, but it is no
substitute for the excitement of the real thing. It is
also—and this is the point—much easier than the
real thing. One can fantasize that one is Jim McMahon
and still be woefully out of shape physically and
unwilling to accept the pain or the possibility of
losing. Every fan in the grandstand can be a great
quarterback in dream life and it requires no discipline, no practice, no suffering at all. Similarly, one
can play with the Playmate of the centerfold without
ever having to practice or suffer the pain and disci-

pline of acquiring skill as an effective player in the sexual game.

All the Playmate has to do is pose and smile. When one has overcome the embarrassment of it, it is a relatively easy task. There is no need to master the skills that the pose and smile imply. The Playmate of the Month looks playful, but in the real world she could be frigid, uninterested in men, terrified of sex, bitchy, or just plain blah in bed. The tease, the pose, the smile of the Playmate may be great for the reader's fantasy life and they may even make some marginal contribution to her own, but they have little relevance for anybody's sex life. It's not the phoniness that bothers us so much—that, after all, is an element in fantasy that concerns itself with the unreal, the puffed up, the make-believe. It is the pretense that this is what play is all about that rings so false.

To be a playmate or to have a playmate is at least as difficult in its own order as being a professional quarterback. There are people who *look* like quarterbacks, but they haven't got what it takes. Strong arms, strong legs they may possess; and with the uniform and equipment they look great on the sports pages. It is not enough to look like a quarterback; one must be one. It is not enough to look like a Playmate; one must be good at playing.

To have a playmate means to be in possession of someone who has made themselves a specialist in your physiology-psychology-fantasy life. It means that you belong to someone who has devoted long years and much practice to understanding you and reading you and is perfectly happy continuing to practice and perfect his skills. It means that you have yielded yourself to the other's power and influence. To permit someone else to be your playmate is a delightful yet terrifying experience. As Martin D'Arcy pointed out long ago, <u>love is not so much possessing as being possessed. Only the brave can permit themselves to be possessed.</u> Your partner becomes the playmate when you have become brave enough to permit that partner to possess you. And when this happens there is no way out of the commitment. The question of the permanency of commitment becomes theoretical and irrelevant. When the kind of possession required for sexual playfulness has occurred, there is no way out; one does not want to get out, and even the thought of it is absurd. There may still be conflict and tension in the relationship; indeed, any relationship between humans will certainly generate some conflict. But being possessed by a playmate also means being obsessed by him (or her).

Sexual playfulness, then, begins in earnest only when one has given oneself to another so totally that there is simply no way back. In the fantasy of playing with the centerfold sex object the emphasis is almost always on what the spectator does to and with the body so invitingly displayed on the foldout. In real life, playfulness means what one is willing to permit the other to do to oneself. The male who indulges in his late adolescent fantasies with Playmate of the Month might very well be paralyzed with terror if the woman whose picture attracts him should stride into his real life and demand the kind of influence, power, and control over him that real-life playmates must have if the game is to begin.

Similarly, the modern liberated woman who joins the growing ranks of those who buy *Playgirl* may shiver with anticipation at the fantasies that arise from the promises of the magazine. But in real life she is most reluctant to yield as much of herself to a man as would be required to make those fantasies anything but daydreams.

Real playmates are scary people, because they want us body and soul. If we give ourselves to them they will indeed provide all the pleasure and happiness they promise, but there will be fear and suffering in the constant struggle to become more fully possessed and to more fully possess. The centerfold characters—male or female—promise everything and demand nothing. Real playmates demand everything, and they are not satisfied until they get it. They learn only slowly and with difficulty how to effectively demand everything from us; and we learn only slowly and with difficulty how to respond to their demands. Both the playmate and the one with whom he (or she) plays acquire the skills of the game only with effort after mistakes, miscues, false starts, and failures.

Having a playmate and being one are reciprocal phenomena. Another person will be a playmate for us to the extent that we are fierce and determined enough to take possession of the other even as he (or she) is possessing us. We must be a specialist in the other's physiology-psychology-fantasy in the same way the other is a specialist in ours. There are no shortcuts, no easy way out, no manuals to explain how to do it, no weekend courses to give us a degree validating our sexual playfulness. A good deal of the coin of the realm can be accumulated by those who write books and run weekend sessions on sex. There is titillation in them and the satisfaction that comes from feeling one is enlightened and a member of the avant-garde—so perhaps those who read and attend get their money's worth. To give the sex manuals and the encounter movement the most I will concede to them, a little bit may happen to those involved in them in a few cases. But, in general, attempts to short-circuit the long, slow, difficult road to possession and being possessed may be fun but they are fundamentally counterfeit. They frequently reinforce the fears, the anxiety, the game playing, the hiding behind masks that enable so many couples to escape the terrors of playing in the sexual game.

One of the principal obstacles to sexual play is the myth of competence. The assumption of the *Playboy* Philosophy and of more sophisticated forms of contemporary hedonism is that the spectator is already competent. Show a man the Playmate of the Month and he knows what to do to her; show a woman the centerfold of *Playgirl* and she knows how to react. Indeed, *Playboy* (and to a lesser and derivative extent *Playgirl*, too) constantly flatters their readers by assuring them of their indubitable, unquestioned sexual omnicompetence. It's nice to be told we're good in bed, because we know we should be but have the sinking feeling that we are not.

Most adults know how babies are born. They know how sexual organs are made to be linked, and under appropriate circumstances they can perform the indicated operation with a certain minimum amount of efficiency. If that were all that is required to be an effective lover, then almost everyone would be sexually competent. Fears of sexual inadequacy that assail most of us would have no meaning at all.

But sex is between people, not merely between bodies. People are different; one can reach orgasm with a prostitute, but one can only play with another human whom he knows. And that brings us up against the mystery of another person's self.

Lock a man in a room with a Playmate of the Month and tell him he must make love to her. He will be sexually aroused, of course, but he will also be terrified because now he faces a real woman—attractive, mysterious, complex, baffling, able to respond at the promptings of herself, not only *his* fantasies. He can force himself crudely and brutally upon her and achieve the basic release that comes from orgasm; but this is not what his masculine ego and self-confidence demand of him. The interlude with this beautiful woman must be an event to remember, not just a few quick physiological spasms. She must enjoy it as much as he does. The totality of both their persons must be involved in a memorable and thoroughly satisfying experience. She is waiting for him to begin. What does she want? How should he start? How should they do it? How long should they prepare? What kind of foreplay would be best? What will really turn her on? What kinds of tenderness and affection will be most reassuring and stimulating? What can he do to make her respect and admire him? How can it be the kind of event that will make her want more of the same? How can he impress her as a sexually imaginative, creative, competent male? It is as though he has been put in the huddle of the Chicago Bears and called upon to deliver the game-winning pass when he can't even remember the game plan. Under such circumstances not a few men would become impotent and many others would simply turn into brutes. They are put into a situation where sexual competence is demanded of them immediately, and they simply do not know what to do.

Put a woman in the same situation where she is imprisoned with an extraordinarily attractive male who makes it perfectly clear that he is willing to make love. In her fantasy life she had dreamed repeatedly of having such a splendid male body available, but now she simply does not know what to do. Does he really find her attractive? Is she too thin or too fat? Are her sex organs too big or too small? Can she really hold his attention and interest? What should they talk about? How should she begin? What should she do with her hands and her mouth? What kinds of things would he like to do to her? Why is she so frightened? Is she frigid?

We feel incompetent with strangers. It may be possible to do the bare minimum, although a man frightened into impotency by a strange encounter may not be able to do even that. Sexual competency is not a generalized ability, save for a few simple and easily learned physiological movements. It is an interpersonal competency gained with this particular person who happens to be our sexual partner at this particular segment of the space-time continuum. The stranger can't be a playmate because he (or she) doesn't know us and we don't know him. An interlude with a stranger may be successful enough to achieve mutual orgasmic release, and there may be a lucky occasion or two when strangers discover important physiological characteristics about one another quickly enough to heighten the pleasure of the experience. But the payoff declines rapidly, because there is far more in sexual play than the tension release of orgasm, however spectacular it may be. The strangers may become playmates, but they do so by exactly the same long, slow process of discovering the totality of one another's selfhood that occurs in any sustained sexual commitment. There is no reason, in other words, why this particular man and this particular woman should expect immediate sexual competency with one another. On the contrary, if they are wise they will expect a lifelong growth in mutual competency. And if they are already well into their marriage, they are simply deceiving themselves if they have become convinced that they are so competent with one another that there is nothing more to learn. Interpersonal sexual competency can be said to only begin when a couple has been together for a considerable amount of time. If we were just animals, that would not be the case. But we are human animals, with fears, anxieties, needs, longings, and, above all, complex systems of meaning that interpret for us all the events of our life, particularly those that challenge us most directly as men and women. The real playmate is one who has achieved a high degree of competency in dealing with us because he (or she) shares our body, our spirit, our fantasy life and our meaning systems. When we are put into a room with such a person and told that we have nothing else to do but make love, questions of competency are quite irrelevant.

Hence the essential prerequisite for growth in playfulness is the admission that we are not competent automatically and that we have to grow and learn what competency means with this other person. It is a hard admission to make, hard at the beginning of marriage and even harder as the years go on. For a man to admit to his wife, "I don't really know you. I don't really know how to make love to you," is a shattering experience. (Of course, it need not be expressed in those words.) For a woman to say to her husband, "You are a mystery to me. I have no real notion of how to please and satisfy you," is also shattering. Such admissions are an acceptance of the necessity for trust, confidence, respect, and affection to be established in some amount at least as an atmosphere conducive to the growth of sexual competence and playfulness. You can only admit that you are *not* good at something in the presence of another who is already sufficiently impressed by you that your admission of incompetence is not likely to diminish his respect for you. One can admit incompetence in most cases only in a set of circumstances where one can be reasonably confident that the other will increase rather than decrease his respect for you precisely because of the admission. If the man is convinced that when he says to his wife that he does not really understand how to make her happy, she will love him more, not less, his concession becomes relatively easy—though still painful. A woman will find it much easier to tell her husband that she needs to know much more about what is required to bring him pleasure (in bed and in the rest of their relationship) if she knows that his love will be deepened by such a request.

In other words, when we admit our lack of competence and our inadequacies in circumstances where there is already love and affection, then we are engaged precisely in that process of self-disclosure and self-revelation that is already erotic play. The confession of inadequacy and the desire to learn is already an act of sexual playfulness—and in the proper circumstances an intensely erotic one. "Show me how" is just about the most seductive thing one can say to his sexual partner, yet the words are so hard to say, they stick so rigidly in our throat.

Playfulness also requires the freedom to learn by mistakes, failures, and trial and error. If the whole relationship depends on the success of every experiment, then playfulness doesn't have much of a life expectancy. A woman reads that a sheer black bra will turn a man on, so she buys the naughtiest one she can find and gives her husband a good, long look at her in it one evening. He seems mildly interested in how much it cost, but is not aroused at all. If he were really sensitive, he would of course catch what she was trying to do and respond enthusiastically, if not to the garment, at least to her. No one is sensitive to every cue all the time. If this failure so discourages the woman that she is unwilling to risk other "naughty" experiments, then there is simply not enough trust and playfulness in the relationship for the awkward trial-and-error growth, which is the only way playfulness can expand and develop.

Similarly, a man finds himself intrigued by what he has heard of some of the "French" techniques of combining lovemaking and powerlessness. He explains the techniques to his wife and she shows a mild interest. They experiment and discover that the experience is considerably less for them than the wild, incredible pleasure the sex manuals promised. Both are bound to be somewhat disappointed, but if they can laugh the incident off and add it to the growing list of shared jokes, the fund of trust and playfulness is great enough for their continued expansion and growth.

Techniques are relatively unimportant when compared with the fundamental dynamics of a relationship. Two human beings living in what is frequently oppressive intimacy make mistakes in dealing with each other every day. A thoughtless word, a joke that is intended to be funny but is cutting and hurtful, a burst of exasperation at the wrong time, a trivial complaint when tenderness is needed—these can either be laughed off or become part of the hidden agenda of frustration, anger, and bitterness. Playfulness in bed and playfulness in the totality of a relationship mutually reinforce one another. Genital sexuality that is rigid and unimaginative inhibits the growth of playfulness in the common life, and a common life that is grim, serious, "responsible," and filled with mistakes, reprimands, and temper tantrums is not going to be transformed into play when the bedroom door closes.

Play is competitive. There is a certain kind of "do-good" mentality in the United States that thinks competition is Capitalist Immorality and that little children should learn to cooperate with one another instead of competing. Competition is part of the vitality of life. Little children compete and cooperate simultaneously in their games. They cannot compete unless they set up a framework of cooperation, and it is the enjoyment and challenge of competition that encourages them to sustain and improve the cooperation that provides the context of the game. What is wrong is the belief that you have to win all the time for the competition to be worth the effort. If the only fun in the game is winning, the game isn't much fun at all. No one can win all the time, and people who equate losing the game with failure in a wider sense miss the point of competition completely. (Incidentally, I find grammar school athletic programs repellent. Pickup contests, sandlot games, ad hoc confrontations on the playing fields are great fun and part of growing up for both boys and girls. Well-organized, uniformed, efficiently coached operations—like Little League, for example—are a serious business and designed more for parents than as healthy sport for children. These contests are so important to the parent because he, having lost all sense of playfulness, equates losing a game with failure in the real world.)

Part of the fun of the game is its competitiveness. "I top you, you top me"; "I'm better than you are, you're better than I am"; "I can do something you can't do, you can do something I can't do." Indeed, the more fiercely competitive the game, the more fun it is for both sides because the more it challenges both to their maximum efforts. Only when the rules of the game are violated and the norms of the outside world are brought in does loss mean failure and defeat mean ignominy. Then, of course, one of the players will end the game and go home.

When a man and woman are cramped together in the narrow life space of their marriage there will be competition and conflict as they spar together for relative advantage over the limited resources that are available to them. Such conflict and competition are a way of working out tensions, of balancing needs, and of strengthening the bonds that hold the joint venture together. If the competition can be approached with the playfulness of the game world, where the competition is real indeed but not "serious" in the sense that the fundamental ego strength and indispensable needs of either partner are being violated, then the bonds of cooperation are strengthened. They *struggle* together in order that they may struggle *together*. They contend with each other the way Jacob did with the angel of Yahweh, not in anger, not to tear the relationship apart, but in order to bind it together more solidly. The wrestling match between Jacob and the angel of Yahweh was indeed a wrestling match. God and Jacob were contending, fighting, competing with one another, but it was a competition that grew out of love and reinforced that love.

Sexual competitiveness is indescribably erotic. If each partner is struggling to be better than the other sexually, it necessarily means that each is struggling to be better at giving pleasure to the other rather than taking it for oneself. It is the kind of competition in which everybody wins. If the husband has a particularly good night, in which his wife is at first reluctant and resistant and ends up almost pathethically pleading for more, he has won but so has she. If the wife drives out of her husband's mind all distractions, all thoughts of other women, indeed everything but desire for her by a scene that will haunt him for several days, she has triumphed indeed, but he has not exactly been a loser. To win a point in the sexual game is an absolute delight. "I showed him" or "I showed her" is a cry of exultation and self-satisfaction, but to lose a point by being shown is also a memorable experience.

Competition in the sexual game becomes unhealthy only under two circumstances: either one of the partners won't play, or one of the partners refuses to let the other play. In both cases all points are scored on one side, and the other is reduced, by his choice or by his partner's, to playing the role of passive cooperator. He becomes a respondent and audience who must react to and applaud the triumphs of the perennial victor. Some men's sexual egos are so weak that this is the only kind of game they are capable of playing. Their relationship with a woman must be an endless series of "scores." Some women are so prudish, so passive, or so frightened that to "win" a sexual tussle with a man would be to deny their own femininity. Such children, the conquering

male and the ever-conquered female, may blend together in a stable relationship, and presumably worse
things could happen to them. The man might have
married a woman who insists on "scoring" sometimes herself, and she might have married a man
who wants to be challenged as well as applauded
and accepted. But such stable, routine, one-way relationships ought not to be confused with playfulness.
Nobody wants to play golf with the pro who shoots
in the low 70s unless he plays with an equalizing
handicap. Sexual competitiveness between a husband and wife enhances the sex gain only when
there is relative equality between the contestants,
which means that the husband must be brave enough
to lose some of the encounters and the wife brave
enough to win some of them.

The very use of the words "win" and "lose" will
be offensive to some. How can one speak of winning
and losing in something as intimate and private as
human love? It is not difficult if one remembers that
in the world of the game one's success or failure as a
human or as a man or woman is in no way connected
to whether one wins or loses the game. The equations winning = success, losing = failure are an
invasion of the world of the game by norms and
values that do not belong there. A husband and wife
involved in a deeply affectionate and playful sexual
relationship with each other will have no problem at
all understanding what I mean. The husband has
many times experienced self-satisfaction, pride, and
complacency as he drops off to sleep thinking, "I
really did it to her tonight," while the wife is falling
asleep happily overwhelmed by an aggressive, demanding, absolutely implacable lover. Tonight she
lost, but she had as much fun losing as he did
winning.

For a woman to think to herself that this was her night for victory may well be even more exciting and rewarding than it would be for her husband. For in the culture in which she was raised, winning in sex is a male prerogative. To be able to win at the game is to show both the culture and her husband. She can be weak, passive, and surrendering when that is appropriate; she can be as fierce, demanding, impassioned, and as implacable as he when that is her mood.

Perhaps the most pleasurable kind of sexual play comes on those occasions when both the man and the woman are in aggressive, implacable moods. The competition then is indeed a fierce fight; it is Jacob wrestling with the angel of Yahweh. The struggle is wild, passionate, terrifying, indescribably enjoyable. Which of the partners "wins" may ultimately depend on the fine-tuned sensitivity of the other. If they are really skillful players at the sexual game they will be able to know when the other really ought to win, when at the last moment one substitutes graceful surrender for continued conflict. This is, of course, sexual playfulness refined to a high art. But the nice thing about having a lifetime playmate is that one has a long time to refine one's skills at the art. The equations of the sexual game may be unique in the game world: losing = winning, winning = winning. That's a game to bet on!

Playmates must be strong. They must refuse to take "no" for an answer (save on those occasions when their sensitivities reveal to them that "no" is reasonable with no diminution of love and trust). The playmate must have the vigor and the resourcefulness to tear away the masks and the defenses, the protections, the phony fears, the silly anxieties—all those escape hatches one uses to flee the terrors and delights of the sexual game. Strength requires confidence, of course, and a playmate who is not confident of his or her abilities to deal effectively with a sexual partner will not be much of a playmate. Conflict can coexist with the admission that one's competency needs to grow and develop. Indeed the assertion of omnicompetence is normally an attempt to hide lack of confidence. The confident playmate says in effect, "There may still be much I have to learn about my spouse's fantasies, needs, desires, responses; but I know enough to be able to begin, and I am secure enough in our relationship to be able to move ahead." Confidence means that one is strong enough, secure enough, and knowledgeable enough to begin, knowing that afterwards the "playing by ear" that inevitably follows will not be a total failure. The problem for the man locked in the room with the Playmate of the Month that we discussed earlier is that he really doesn't know how to begin. How can he, since he is dealing with a stranger? Surely the first time a couple who have committed themselves to each other come together they too lack confidence, but they can both feel brave enough, strong enough, secure enough, accepted enough, loved enough to begin. Competency grows when confidence is a given.

But it is a given that needs constant reinforcement. If we expect our sexual partner to become a playmate for us, we must constantly support, reinforce, and build the partner's ego strength. A man needs to be told day in and day out that he is a good lover—even on those occasions when he is only adequate. A woman needs to hear, in season and out, that she is a totally gorgeous, desirable, seductive, irresistible female—even on those occasions when her awkwardness and hesitance make her quite resistible. A partner becomes a playmate to the extent that we successfully define him (or her) as such. A man cannot hear too often from his wife that she wants his body in hers; and she cannot hear too often from him that her breasts are so delectable that he simply cannot keep his hands off them.

To what extent must this pursuit of confidence and competence be explicit for the sexual game to flourish? Is it an art that can be pursued implicitly, tacitly, unreflectively? Or must it be something that is the subject of constant explicit dialogue and discussion within a relationship?

There are no clear and simple answers to these questions. Some people can develop an extraordinarily playful sexual relationship through skilled communication that is almost always subliminal and unobtrusive. Others can become easy and matter-of-fact in discussing the most intimate details of their lovemaking. Still others talk about it constantly, persuading themselves and boring others about their really great sex life when in fact they are blindly following the paradigms they find in the most recent manual. Finally, some people may be so tied in puritanical knots that they pretend most of the time that no such thing as sex exists in their life together. The style with which a couple pursues mastery of sexual playfulness depends upon the style of their personalities and the style of their relationship. Some talk too much, others not nearly enough. On balance it can be said that for most American couples the real risk is that they will not talk nearly enough.

To be "masterful" (or "mistressful") at the sexual game is to be in command of the situation, to be able to combine implacable firmness with sensitive tenderness, to know when to comfort, when to challenge, when to insist, when to defer, when to push, when to yield, when to become angry, when to reassure, when to win, when to lose, when to overwhelm, when to be overwhelmed, when to tear away resistance, and when to respect it. One can only learn these delicate arts by experimentation, practice, and attention to feedback. In the ordinary course of events most human beings gain mastery only to the extent that they focus self-conscious energy and effort on the process. It is not something that comes easily, naturally, or unreflectively.

To the argument that there are too many other obligations and responsibilities and important things in life to devote time to such a frivolous pursuit, one can only say that this is an option some people freely choose, but it is one that, in principle at least, is an obligation for no one. It may well be that there are other satisfactions in life that make sexual playfulness seem relatively unimportant. If that is the case for a given couple, so be it; but they are kidding themselves if they think that they have rejected an option that did not contain pleasure, variety, wonder, and reward. It is a good thing to be masterful, to feel that one has supreme and loving power over the other, that one can possess the other without his or her having the ability or the desire to resist. It is also good to know that one is under such tender but effective domination by another human being, that there is someone who can do with us whatever he or she wants, and that whatever he or she wants is what we want. Those who don't particularly care for such payoffs in their lives are within their rights in rejecting them, but they can scarcely dismiss as fools those who think otherwise.

A man puts his arm around his wife. She is limp, weary, depressed, and reluctant; it has been a hard day for her. His personality expands, blood rushes through his veins, his heart stirs because he knows that he has within himself the power to bring that limp body alive with pleasure and delight. It is not an absolutely necessary thing for a man to have such an experience, but it is a good thing, and for most men the more often they can have it, the better.

A woman sees her husband's face lined with care and preoccupation. There are a thousand and one troubled, anxious thoughts darting through his mind. She slips off her dress and exults in the power that is hers to so transform things that in a few moments there will be only one thing on his mind. When she is finished with him, the world will necessarily be brighter and warmer and more benign. It is not necessary for a woman to experience such exultation in her womanliness. Still it doesn't hurt, and most women cannot experience it too often. Playfulness, then, is not indispensable, but the question is, why should anyone want to dispense with it?

To be playful in a sustained sexual relationship means to keep romance alive. Romance requires imagination, sympathy, understanding, persistence, sensitivity. It also requires physical tenderness. The frequency with which people make love depends on their tastes and needs. (Nine times a month is the American average, we are told.) But if physical tenderness is limited to just lovemaking, there is little romance left in the relationship. There are many times in the course of a life together when a gentle touch, a quick caress, a light kiss convey more passion, more romance, more commitment, and more playfulness than an extended romp in bed. The essence of playfulness is not so much that there is a necessity to do anything, but that there is an opportunity to do practically everything. Probably it is that absence of obligation and the presence of unlimited opportunity in sexual playfulness that most offends the puritans.

16

It ought to be easy to write about sexual fantasies. Everyone has them, and some are extremely vivid sexual daydreams. They have been the basis of all pornography and much great art, music, and literature (implicitly if not explicitly) in the course of human history. The current merchandisers of sexual fantasy show surprisingly little sophistication compared with many of their predecessors. As camera work, the photographs in *Playboy* may be excellent, but the fantasy they evoke is crude, gross, and unimaginative. It may appeal to the adolescent segment of the fantasy spectrum, but not to the more mature, nuanced, and subtle fantasy lives of which even *Playboy* addicts are capable. Read, for example, Joseph Conrad's description of lust in his *Outcast of the Islands* and compare it with a *Playboy* centerfold and decide which is more erotic.

But if sexual fantasy is universal, appealing, and powerful, it is also a very awkward subject for discussion. Most people are ashamed of their fantasies, or they do not understand them. Many feel so guilty about them that they must vigorously deny them and launch angry attacks on those who hint of their existence. Some of the opposition to pornography, for example, is probably based on guilt about one's own vivid imagination. It seems that sexual fantasy is a subject that cannot be discussed coolly and dispassionately. Most of the systematic study and knowledge about fantasy life comes either from the psychiatrist's couch or from nonrandom and not necessarily representative interviews. We know only our own fantasies and are reluctant to believe that other people may have the same images in their imaginations. Psychologists understand very dimly the purpose and functioning of human fantasy life—sexual or otherwise—although they agree that it is the source of art, poetry, and religious symbols and it is of critical importance in the development of both human personality and human social culture.

Our fantasy lives are wild, disordered, chaotic. To speak of them in any systematic fashion is to impose an order and organization on them that is totally absent in reality. The fantasy world is infantile. It is, to use Norman O. Brown's phrase, "polymorphously perverse." It draws the line at no sexual behavior, because it has not learned like the ego that certain kinds of sex are destructive of human relationships, human society, human civilization. Incest, rape, homosexuality, bestiality, sadomasochistic orgies are all completely undifferentiated in the raw and primal imagination.

Contrary to Professor Brown I do not believe that the polymorphously perverse infantile sexual imagination can be taken as a norm for adult life. The human race turned polymorphously perverse would quickly extinguish itself. Nonetheless we must cope with our sexual fantasies. They are part of the ambiguity of the human condition. The strain between polymorphous perversity and mature self-restraint is one of the most fundamental of ambiguities. Neither of these polarities can be eliminated without destroying the personality.

Are sexual fantasies evil? As fantasies, surely not; they are the natural activity of the imagination of incarnate sexual beings. They become evil when we attempt to actually accomplish all of them (which happens usually only among the unbalanced), or when we permit them to substitute for relationships in the world occupied by real human beings. Some fantasies can be carried out into the real world; other fantasies give us critical hints about our personality and our needs; and still others can provide a richness and variety in our sexual relations that may substantially improve our emotional life and our psychological well-being. Finally, sexual fantasy has profoundly religious overtones. It is part of the preconscious self that produces both sexual and religious images, which are inextricably linked in many cases in the same symbol.

Such a suggestion is offensive to puritans. How can something as filthy as "dirty thoughts" be religious? The God that made us with a wild, uncontrollable fantasy life obviously made an artistic mistake. He made an even greater mistake when he permitted the preconscious, from which the grossest sexual images emerge, to also produce the most elevated religious symbols.

To add to the complexities of attempting to discuss sexual fantasies and their role in the relationship between husband and wife, it is impossible to discuss fantasies without describing them. Such descriptions are necessarily erotic, and the pages on which they are written have a tendency to get steamy. Both the puritan and the prurient (and puritans are usually cryptoprurients) can't get beyond the steam. I hasten to add that the fantasies presented in this chapter are tame. Any reader who claims that he or she does not have such fantasies (indeed some that are much wilder) is simply not telling the truth (or perhaps not admitting it to himself or herself).

Despite the complexities of discussing sexual fantasies, the discussion must take place. They are part of the human condition, and to pretend they are not is to ignore the facts. They are part of human sexuality, and an attempt to provide meaning for human sexuality that passes over them is bound to be inadequate. They tell us something critical about the nature and destiny of humankind, and a theology that ignores such data is a theology with blinkers on.

I will confine my discussion to heterosexual fantasies because for most people they are by far the most frequent and because they are the most pertinent to the subject of marriage and sexual play. To wrestle with other kinds of fantasies would take us far afield and muddy even more a complex and intricate subject. Still it must be noted in passing that a mature person knows that sexuality is a continuum and not a sharp dichotomy. A sexually mature man is confident enough in his own maleness that he does not have to try to hide from himself that he sometimes finds the bodies of other men in a shower room sexually appealing. Nor need a woman feel that she is perverted because she occasionally feels a strong urge to play with the breasts of another woman. Such feelings, longings, urges are normal statistically and psychologically. To acknowledge them is merely to concede the complexity of human sexuality. Mature heterosexuals do not take such urges as a norm for action; they do not feel constrained to give in to such longings, and they are not shaken by insecurity or guilt simply because they discover such desires in themselves.

As far as one can judge from the sparse, confused, and uneven psychiatric and social scientific literature on the subject, there are four general kinds of frequent sexual fantasies. Each is as prevalent in men as in women, although they may take different forms in the different sexes.

1. *Fantasies of nakedness.* Dressing and undressing is a primordial human behavior that is filled with sexual implications and overtones beginning with the very earliest childhood memories. To be exposed is to be seen, enjoyed, possessed. Clothes are designed both to conceal and to reveal, to hide and to display. The sexual implications of clothes are so obvious that one should not have to mention it. But the very hint that dressing and undressing are highly sexual activities is enough to send puritans into paroxysms of anger.

Indeed the sexual power of taking off and putting on clothes is so great that lovers in a sustained relationship must develop a (usually) implicit agreement as to when such activity may be permitted to be overtly sexual and when the sexual content of it will be ignored. Otherwise they would be late for every appointment that they had to keep together. Such a modus vivendi may deprive dressing and undressing of any explicit connotation, and undressing may become as casual and insignificant as turning on the TV set. A good criterion of the playfulness of a sexual relationship is the richness, the excitement, the significance that a husband and wife permit the ordinary but highly charged activity of putting on and taking off clothes to be. It is a behavior that is inherently playful with an almost limitless variety of playful possibilities. When all play is gone out of it, there can be little play left in the relationship. If the nightly ritual has become routine in the real world, undressing or being undressed is still pure terror and pure delight in the world of dream and fantasy.

2. *Ravishing and being ravished.* I hesitate to use the word, because ravishing is a sordid, violent, ugly, vicious act. It may occasionally be that in fantasy life too, but fantasy ravishing is transformed and has little in common with the ugly violation of another human being that occurs all too frequently in the real world. For it is of the essence of fantasy ravishing that one is forced to do something that one desperately wants to do, or that one forces the other to do something that the other deeply wants to do. There may be violence in fantasy ravishing but not violation. One may be powerless (or render another powerless), but it is a pleasurable and not a brutalized powerlessness. The essence of fantasy ravishing is that resistance, inhibition, hesitancy are firmly and completely swept away. One either becomes powerless and is completely at the whim of the other or renders the other powerless and has complete control of him (or her).

3. *Seduction and being seduced.* Ravishing fantasies concentrate on the direct, forcible, and, if need be, violent reduction of resistance. Seduction fantasies focus on the slow, gentle art of taking possession of or being possessed by the other. Instead of the process's being quick, firm, even harsh, it is long, teasing, and leisurely. The end is the same, of course, but

the important fact of the imagery is not the end but the style, the modality. In both the rape and seduction fantasies one conquers or is conquered. In the former one's competency is directed at immediate conquest, in the latter it is directed at slow, gradual, agonizingly delightful surrender.

4. *Fantasies that have to do with variety of position, place, and organs involved.* Given that there is an almost limitless variety of places where sex can occur and a considerable number of positions and techniques for obtaining sexual satisfaction with one's partner, there are countless possibilities for fantasies on this subject. Most marital sex takes place in one position, in one place, and with one technique, but this does not prevent the imagination from contemplating a wide variety of interesting possibilities.

Such a list of fantasies is bound to be inadequate and incomplete, but to sketch some of the fantasies that are apparently so frequent as to be universal may tell us something extremely important about human sexuality.

Let us now consider the fantasies of a relatively typical (composite) upper-middle-class American couple. I wish to emphasize that these fantasies are "normal" both in the statistical sense of being commonplace and in the psychological sense of not indicating emotional disturbance. On the contrary, such fantasies (or fantasies like them) are typical to the point of being almost universal among physically healthy adults.

The wife imagines herself being brought to a party of her husband's friends. The men are all wearing evening clothes, and she is wearing a black strapless gown and black lace underthings. Her husband begins to describe quite clinically her sexual attributes. His friends demand evidence and he compels her to slowly remove her clothes. He makes appropriate descriptive comments as she undresses, and his friends applaud in appreciation. Completely naked, she is then compelled to walk among the men while they touch and caress her, leaving not a part of her body untouched. Finally, her husband makes love to her while his friends cheer them on. Her fantasy ends as he turns her over to one of his friends for his pleasure.

The husband is on an airplane on a business trip. He is seated next to an attractive, extremely shapely woman with pale white skin, dark hair turning slightly gray, and a deep seductive voice. In his fantasy she strikes up a conversation, letting her hand wander to his thigh and leaning her body suggestively against his. As they get off the airplane, she invites him to her hotel room. In the room he becomes completely passive and she assumes control of the situation, teasing him to uncontrollable desire. She then kneels astride him and screams with joy as she brings the two of them to a dazzling climax. (In the real world, of course, she gets off the plane without saying a word.)

The wife is in the kitchen finishing up the dishes in early afternoon. She imagines a man entering the room. He is dark, muscular, hard, and clad only in a scanty loincloth. Without saying a word he comes up behind her and locks his arms around her in a fierce embrace. She tries to break away, but her struggles are useless. He kisses the back of her neck and her shoulders, squeezes her breasts, and tightens his grip of her. She stops struggling. Still silent, he unzips her dress, tears away her panties and bra, and forces himself into her—quickly, skillfully, and insistently.

She had never before responded so completely and totally to a man. She is utterly helpless and totally transformed. She can almost feel his hot breath on her face when the phone rings and brings her out of her daydream.

Her husband is having lunch by himself. The waitress is young, pretty, with an air of intelligence and good breeding. He imagines waiting for her after work and inviting her for a drink. They have a fascinating and very intellectual conversation—as well as several drinks. They drive to a deserted place and he begins to kiss and caress her. She resists, pleads with him to stop, but he gets his mouth on her nipple and then his penis between her thighs. She surrenders, giving herself to him completely and totally. Her body responds to his as a custom-made glove fits her hand. On the way back to the city she clings to him and makes him promise that he will do it to her again. In the real world he pays his check, leaves an extra large tip, and departs.

His wife is on the beach, watching the children play near the water. The bronzed young lifeguard is the only other adult in sight. In fantasy the children leave and she approaches the young man. He nervously keeps his eyes away from her as they talk. Her hand rests on his knee and then slides up to his trunks. He looks up at her, a mixture of fear and longing in his eyes. Her lips meet his just as she unhooks the top of her swimming suit. Their two bodies merge on the sand as the waters of the lake wash over them. One of the children intrudes into the daydream with a demand for a drink of water.

Her husband is having a Scotch in the golf course locker room, waiting for his foursome partners to finish their showers. In fantasy he sees through the wall into the women's shower room. He is then dragged into the locker room and pinned against the wall by a group of women in various advanced stages of undress. At the direction of a tall, athletic woman with large breasts and leopard-skin shorts, they take off his clothes and tie him to a bench. The woman all gather round, playing with him, kissing him, pinching him, tickling him, making fun of him. They push their breasts against his lips and make him suck on them; they take turns lying on top of him. Finally they drag him into the shower and have a merry time covering him with soapsuds and hugging and embracing his now wet and slippery body. Before the fantasy goes any further (and he is perfectly pre-pared to go on and on with it) the friends arrive and the post-golf poker game begins.

Note well that we are dealing with two responsi-ble, self-possessed adults. They are good parents, good spouses. The husband would no more attack the young waitress than he would jump off the top of a building. The wife would no more put her hand on the lifeguard's sexual organs than she would put it in a fire. They are not sick or dirty people. Their fantasies—vivid, exciting, and compelling—come out of their experiences and imaginations and are stored up in their unconscious and preconscious minds. If they were hypnotized (which is in itself another fantasy) and compelled to live out their fantasies, they would find it a delightful experience (who wouldn't?) only because they could then be dispensed from freedom of choice, responsibility, and guilt. They are much like the young man in Eric Rohmer's *Chloe in the Afternoon*. In his fantasy life he had a secret power that forced every woman he wanted to bed down with him instantly. But when the very real Chloe became available to him, he fled in panic to return to his wife—who, Rohmer skillfully hints, had fled herself from a similar fantasy turned disturbingly real.

What then are fantasies besides entertaining ways of passing the time? They are first of all a way to release emotional and psychic energy, dangerous only if they become so compulsively important that real human relationships and responsibilities are ignored, or if one seriously begins to turn the fantasies into reality. Daydreams probably have a function not unlike real dreams: They are a harmless way of discharging certain kinds of pent-up energy. In order for the personality to develop a firm core, for society to protect its culture and structure, for human civilization to survive, humankind must learn to divert, channel, restrain, and focus its raw, primal energies. These energies do not go away. In principle we would still like to be able to make love to everyone we find desirable (which, it turns out, includes a very substantial number of potential partners). In practice this is not possible, and we would be afraid of it if it were, but our polymorphously perverse infantile libido is still there and finds outlets for its longings in images, dreams, and fantasies.

But these fantasies also reveal to us—if we are not ashamed to consider their implications—that we are creatures with powerful, deep, complex hungers. We can restrain and control these hungers, but we cannot eliminate them completely and it is a mistake to try. Intimate relationships exist, from one point of view, as safety-valve mechanisms in which some of the raw force of our primal hunger can be discharged in a context of safety and support. Sexual intimacy creates a context in which some of the energy of our sexual fantasy lives can be expended in safe and constructive ways. The more relaxed and playful the intimacy, the easier it is to let the fantasy imp out of the bottle sometimes. In such circumstances the imp not only does not destroy the relationship but enhances it. Intimacy releases fantasy; fantasy reinforces intimacy.

The matron on the beach yearns in fantasy to hold and caress and kiss the penis of the young lifeguard. Indeed, if she is able to be frank with herself, there are many, many penises that she would like to kiss. That obviously is not to be, but her husband's sexual organs are available to be kissed whenever she wishes. He is not likely to mind, or if he prudishly resists at first she can overcome his reluctance. There is no reason why she cannot hold and kiss him every day even if they do not make love. It is not necessary that she do so, of course, but the option is available to her. Out of fear or uncertainty or shame, she may not try; she may even resist when he urges her. No one would argue that the marriage is endangered or that the sexual relationship is no good. The point is that there are a host of ways in which a woman can act out some of her fantasies in a playful relationship with her husband if she wants to do so. To systematically reject all these possibilities is to lock up raw energies that might be constructively and healthily released. There are other ways to release such energies (and celibates can constructively focus them in other directions). Still, for sexual partners it seems foolish not to exploit the potentiality for focusing fantasy energy in exciting, challenging, and delightful playfulness.

Her husband was delighting in his women's-shower-room fantasy until the poker game began. In the unlikely eventuality that a couple of women actually would drag him into a shower, he would be acutely embarrassed. Chances are that his fantasy will not come true, but a warm, soapy, stimulating shower with his wife is another matter altogether. She might resist at first, but if he is afraid to ask, afraid to try, afraid to insist (as many men are), then an opportunity for playfulness that would creatively release some of his fantasy energy has been passed by. The marriage won't end; he may not even be sexually frustrated; but a marriage composed entirely of such missed opportunities will become dull precisely because there is so little emotional energy invested in it.

Fantasy, then, does not provide a detailed outline for reality, but it does open up some interesting possibilities. What possibilities will be pursued depends on the people involved. In the nature of things some relationships can only sustain a relatively limited amount of fantasy discharge and sharing. For either partner to push beyond what the traffic will bear is unwise. On the other hand, some couples can develop a very full, elaborate, and detailed mutual fantasy life. On balance, there is probably room in most relationships for more shared fantasy than actually exists.

To what extent can one share fantasies with another? Some fantasies are intensely private and simply can't be shared. Others can be shared or not, depending on the state of the relationship. Others can be shared with relative ease. There are no hard-and-fast rules; so much depends on the taste, the sense of humor, the self-possession, the emotional strength of the people involved. Certainly the direct encounter group strategy of "Let's sit down now and communicate with each other about our fantasy lives. You tell me yours, and I'll tell you mine" is both foolish and harmful. Fantasies are more likely to be shared in slow gradual self-revelation as a total relation grows in trust and expands in affection. To make them a primary, explicit, and direct item on the mutual agenda is not likely to serve much purpose. Sharing fantasies is no magical cure for a relationship that has serious problems. It is more likely to be an addition to a relationship that is healthy and developing.

Some couples may elaborate several separate fantasy worlds that they can explore together—Turkish harem, Greek slave market, Roman bath, etc. Others may find such highly developed shared fantasies bizarre and kinky. For still others the fantasy sharing may be rather limited and implicit but still important. One husband discovered mostly by guesswork that his wife had a thing about men unbuttoning her blouse. When she wore a blouse it was usually a sign that she was sexually hungry, a sign of which she was unaware. His rather acute sensitivities had picked it up and, although he never talked to her about it, he became quite practiced at unbuttoning blouses, doing so in many unusual places despite some initial resistance on her part. It was a small skill and a small sharing of imagination carried on at a low level of explicit communication. It did not transform the relationship; it did not save the marriage from any threat; but it did make their life together somewhat more playful, and it did improve somewhat the quality of their life together. In all human relationships, however, the "somewhat" may turn out to be cumulatively more important than the big breakthroughs.

I must emphasize that fantasy sharing is an option, not an obligation. There is no all-purpose formula for what ought to be shared or how. Given the fact that most people are so ashamed and so guilty about their fantasy lives, it is likely that fantasy sharing in most relationships will be minimal. I would be suspicious, indeed, of those who contend that they have a great big and very easy fantasy-sharing thing going. My inclination would be to suspect that there is something profoundly wrong with the marriage and the huge fantasy success is a cover-up. Slow, gradual, tasteful, witty sharing of daydreams is probably a sign of a healthy development. Anything else ought to be considered dubious.

Still the daydreams are there, and while we do not act on all of them, they are a relatively important part of our lives. They reveal the variety, the depth, the confusion, the complexity, the passion, the longing of our personalities. They provide some outlet for our psychic energies, they enrich our lives, and, although they may also occasionally drive us to distraction, they frequently provide the raw material for deepening and strengthening long-term sexual commitments. Some of us can use them as the source for artistic creation, and all of us use them for consolation, support, and strengthening the ego.

There are two critical conclusions to be drawn from our reflections about sexual fantasies. First of all, no one is dull. The imagination is active, ingenious, creative, energetic. If we are dull in our sexual relations and in the totality of our lives it is because we repress the variety and ingenuity of our imaginations. Dullness is something that is chosen and accepted, not something built into our natures and personalities. Only when the fantasy world has been completely suppressed does dullness become a chronic affliction.

Finally, the polymorphous perversity of our imagination reveals us as creatures hungering for the absolute in fulfillment and love. Not to be able to make love to everyone we would like to is a frustration for a being who yearns for the Ultimate in possession and being possessed. The infantile primordial energies stirring up constantly in our ids represent the longing of the human spirit to break out of the constraints and limitations that separate it from the rest of the cosmos and to find loving, consuming union with all that is and All That Is. The man who imagines himself being played with in the women's locker room is at a deep psychological level yearning to be played with once again by his mother. But at an even deeper existential level he is yearning for union through surrender to the ultimate maternal power of the universe. The woman lusting for the body of the young lifeguard may be psychologically seeking for the sexual organs of her father, but existentially she is seeking to possess and be possessed by the ultimate paternal power of the universe. Our fantasy life reveals the deep wound in the human personality that was created by our being surrendered in existence as beings who are not Being. But it is through that wound that Being returns with the offer of love and unity.

Thus when a man and woman who are committed to developing a sustained sexual intimacy with each other begin to share their fantasies, they are at the same time sharing their own longings for ultimate union, which in the Christian perspective is Ultimate Union.

What the world of the resurrection will be like we do not know. We used to write off as heathen foolishness the Islamic vision of a paradise of sensual delights. But that vision may not be without insight. That loving unity toward which our sexual fantasies awkwardly grope will be enjoyed in the world of the resurrection. Will it be different from

our imaginings? Surely. But it will be different because it will be better.

Eye has not seen nor ear heard, nor has it entered
into the heart of man....

17

Sexual play is not only fantastic it is also festive. In the early stages of humankind there was but one thing to be celebrated: life itself. Our hold on life then was precarious, but because of our marvelous technological powers we modernists are not aware of how tenuous our hold on life still is and how remarkable is the miracle of daily survival. Our ancestors could not afford the illusion that the survival of life was commonplace.

And so they celebrated each new evidence that in the struggle between order and chaos, between life and death, life and order had won another round. The festivals were festivals of life, of the birth of young animals, of the first fruits, of harvest, of vintage, of planting, of the returning sun in its annual circuit from north to south. (The Jewish Passover feast, become the Christian Easter, was a spring fertility festival. The paschal lamb represented the first fruit of the flocks, and the unleavened bread, the first fruit of the fields. Christmas, the feast of light, replaced the pagan feast of the return of the sun. The Ember Days, those pagan residuals of an era when man was closer to nature, represented feasts of planting, first fruits, harvest, and vintage. Memorial Day, Labor Day, Thanksgiving may be rough secular equivalents.) When the young animals were born, the first fruits harvested, the grapes picked, our primitive ancestors felt that they were participating in and continuing the primal conflict between life and death, between order and chaos, which occurred at the beginning of the cosmos and from which the ordered world had taken its beginning. The spring festival and the harvest festival were profoundly religious celebrations of life. In such celebrations our ancestors united themselves with the gods and their battle against chaos, sought the gods' blessing on their work, and perhaps also passed on to their children the secret lore of the field and the flocks. For since planting and tilling and bringing to harvest were religious activities, so the knowledge of how this ought to be done was religious too.

In these celebrations, sex and religion were mixed so as to be indistinguishable. The festivals were festivals of life and fertility, and of course the most powerful life force in themselves and in other creatures that humans knew was sex. It was fertility that continued the flocks, reproduced the fields each year, and kept their own clan or tribe or village going even when individuals died. Sex was evidently, indisputably sacred. Sacred celebrations then were necessarily sexual.

The orgy of the Roman Saturnalia (which we keep alive if not at Christmas then surely at New Year) was merely a late and secularized version of the primitive notion that on feasts when life was celebrated one should let all the forces of life run wild and free. Sexual abandon at the time of celebration was a way of celebrating and a way of uniting oneself with the powerful life forces. Sexual intercourse in the newly planted fields was a magical attempt to link the fundamental life forces of the universe with the life of the tribe and the village and its crops. There is some evidence that in remote parts of European mountain regions (Spain, France, Yugoslavia, Italy, Hungary) the custom of intercourse in the fields survived even into the first part of this century. Archaic people, who viewed all of life as organic, did not draw sharp distinctions between the fertility of their own bodies and that of their fields; they were both part of the fundamental life-giving force of the cosmos.

That sex was celebration and that celebration was sexual was so self-evident to archaic people that they would not even have thought to question it.

I know of one young man who was blessed with the splendid nickname Spuds. His parents in an outburst of playfulness uncharacteristic of their people had deliberately and consciously decided that he ought to be conceived in a potato field in Ireland. How his nickname will be explained to Spuds when he begins to ask where he got it is a problem for his parents to contend with. (Recently, many years after I wrote that last sentence—which they read—Spuds's parents insisted that I ask him the question. Me: "Spuds, where did you get that nickname?" Spuds (now a teenager): "I was conceived in a potato field in Ireland [big grin]. That's why I'm so cool!" Doubtless.)

Civilization, technology, puritanism, Enlightenment, rationality have all but broken this organic thread of life celebration. Even if we repair that thread and begin to see that our food, our bodies, our cosmos all emerge from one supremely powerful life-giving process we would do so self-consciously, reflectively, deliberately. There are advantages to that, of course. Unlike our primitive ancestors we can reflect on and understand more deeply these primal unions. We can express them not only in music, art, poetry, and dance but also in philosophy, theology, and social science. We have paid for our sophistication by falling from a certain level of innocence, and by its very nature reflection makes us self-conscious and deprives us of unsophisticated spontaneity.

Sex, for our archaic ancestors, was necessarily public. There was no way the life-giving forces could be hidden, covered, prettied up. Sexual intercourse even among primitive peoples usually took place in some sort of privacy (though it meant something different to them than to us, no doubt). But conception and reproduction were public events fraught with powerful and deeply religious implications. Public or quasi-public intercourse on great religious feasts served to remind the members of the tribe that sexual relationships were not just personal, private affairs to be carried out between men and women in carefully secluded secrecy. It prolonged the existence of the tribe and united it with the basic creative processes of the cosmos. Sex was both a celebration and an event to be celebrated.

Mind you, all of this was ritualistic and objective. Sexual play and celebration were enacted in song and dance, the basic parameters of which were very carefully regulated by the historic traditions. The internal selves of the people involved in the ritual were not necessarily affected. One engaged in festive behavior and was perhaps carried away by it to experience it deeply and internally, but it was a very unselfconscious form of personal involvement. No more was required or possible, because the person was not sharply distinct from the rest of the organism that was the village or the tribe. The question of whether the sexual play that was part of the religious celebration was self-fulfilling or not would have been totally meaningless to primitive celebrants. It would never have occurred to them to ask whether "I'm getting anything out of this celebration."

A man and woman engaging in intercourse in a field they had just planted may have enjoyed the experience above and beyond what was required by the ritual. But the game was played according to its rubrics whether they personally felt playful or not. Indeed, their own internalized playfulness was scarcely to the point. In the objective order their sexual play was far more developed than our own, but subjective playfulness could easily be minimal and indeed it was neither required nor understood. If one unselfconsciously intuits the connections between all life-giving forces, then the abandonment of oneself to the interplay of those forces is equally unselfconscious. Subjective play may not have been possible in those archaic societies, but then it was not necessary. In our own age, playfulness is either subjectively enjoyed or we do not define it as play at all. On the whole I think this is progress, but it is progress that makes life far more complicated.

Compare the farmer and his wife copulating in the field in order to keep the ancient ritual magic alive with Spuds's parents in the rain-soaked potato field—I presume it was rain-soaked; Ireland is always rain-soaked. The former couple continue the ancient practice they do not understand and on which they do not reflect, because of a desperate hope that their actions will improve the chances of a good crop, on which their lives, or at least their prosperity, depend. The latter are engaging in an act of pure merriment, not to say devilment. It seems to be simply a hell of a lot of fun to conceive your first child in a potato field in the land of his predecessors. Both couples are keeping a tradition alive, one objectively and unselfconsciously, the other subjectively and unselfconsciously in a burst of euphoria. We self-conscious moderns have a difficult time getting into the heads of the farmer and his wife, but we have little trouble understanding Spuds's parents. We may think they're crazy; we may envy them; but we certainly know what they are up to.

One of the differences between us and our archaic ancestors is that for all our talk about sexual permissiveness and openness we have privatized and profaned sex. Intercourse is now something that takes place between two human beings without any implications for anyone else in the society. What they do is their business (unless they are contributing to the population explosion). It is an event that may have deep meaning for them, but it has no particular meaning for the rest of us. Indeed, there is no direct way they can share it with us, especially when a child does not result from their union—and nowadays children result only in carefully regulated numbers. Society truly does not intrude on their sex life the way it used to. There is also no way their sex life can be related to the rest of humankind. Privatism is a two-edged sword: It protects you from outside intrusion but prohibits you (at least inhibits you) from sharing. Unprivatized sex may be part of celebrations, even religious celebrations. It may become part of public play, albeit highly objectified and ritualized play. Privatized sex does not participate in public celebrations and is sharply separated from

religious ritual. It is very difficult for privatized sex
to maintain its festive and celebratory characteristics. Hence, of course, it becomes profane. We may
sacralize the sexual union with a marriage ceremony
and perhaps frequent renewals of the marriage vows,
but the sacred is invoked in these ways to create a
distant and legalistic context. It does not represent
the life-giving powers of the cosmos and does not
permeate in awe and mystery the ongoing union
between man and woman. Sex is no longer part of
public celebration. Nor is it set in a context of sacred
and religious festivity. The man and woman have
been freed from the ties of both church and state,
tribe and cult. What they do now is their own business; only, unfortunately, desacralized, privatized sex
can easily become dull, uneventful, and monotonous.
The web of meaning that supported sex in its objective playfulness has been sundered. The burden, then,
is almost entirely on the man and woman themselves to create a web of meaning of their own, in
which subjective playfulness can grow and in which
sexual celebration can survive when it is enjoyed
subjectively.

The problem is yet to be considered seriously.
Some free-love communards and other counterculture
types have tried to re-create the fluidity and the
dynamism of archaic sexual celebration, as though
one could instantaneously and by freely chosen social contract reconstruct the archaic world, which
has been irrevocably lost. Many men and women
have their own "mini celebrations" in which birth-
days, anniversaries, special commemorations become
occasions for special and more elaborate sexual interchanges. A few couples set aside a day, a night,
or a weekend a couple of times a year for their own
very private and very much do-it-yourself "ember

day." There are also certain days during the year—particularly, I suspect, Christmas and New Year's Eve—when the atmosphere of sexual encounter between husband and wife is deliberately and self-consciously transformed. In this way one may involve oneself in a celebration that is widespread and public, but it must be noted that all of these sexual celebrations are optional and it is up to the individual couple to decide whether they will occur or not or whether they are celebratory or not. Finally, the notion that lovemaking unites the couple not only with each other but with the rest of humankind and with the fertility of the cosmos—a notion that was so obvious and unquestionable to our ancestors—rarely even occurs to contemporary men and women.

Play is festive by its very nature. It is enjoyable; it is a celebration of human strength, dignity, and integrity, an affirmation that human creative forces can triumph over disorder, confusion, and death. Sociologist Peter Berger quite properly points out that play is a "rumor of angels," "a hint of the transcendent," a signal of what the universe means, a blunt, brilliant, brave affirmation on the part of humankind that death will not snuff out our dazzling creativity. The player, like the unconscious, is confident of his own immortality. In the world of play he shuts out as unreal the thought of death, of nothingness, of oblivion.

The game is serious, but it is not deadly serious. On the contrary it is vitally serious, because the game is a celebration of life over death. Play that is not celebratory is just not play; and sex without a celebratory dimension will become grim, somber, and deadly serious. For a man and woman sex will become a celebration or it can never be playful.

But what is there to celebrate? This is unfortunately a question that all too many married people ask with deadly seriousness. We celebrate the fact that we are alive; that we can eat and drink, sleep and wake, and make love; that we have family and friends; that the sun rises, the moon shines, the rain falls, the sky is blue; that there is food to eat and wine (beer, vodka, gin, Scotch, Irish mist, bourbon, etc., etc.) to drink. We celebrate the good times together and our surviving the bad times, the mistakes we have learned from, the growth we have experienced, the joy and the delight and the pleasure we are able to take in one another's bodies.

The demanding, responsible routine of upper-middle-class professional lives leaves us little time to enjoy, little time to realize that there are things to be enjoyed, and practically no time to celebrate that which we have enjoyed. Can one imagine anything less celebratory than a suburban Christmas cocktail party? The light of the world has come indeed!

Sex, then, is a celebration of both its own over-whelming pleasure and power and all the other good things that the powers of light and life have made available to us. When someone says that he or she is too tired or too worn out at the end of the day to have anything to celebrate, it may well be that the absolute truth is spoken. But this is not a judgment on the things in the universe that ought to be celebrated or on the celebratory power of sexual intercourse. It is merely a reflection on how oppressingly, stultifyingly dull the person has permitted his (or her) life to become. If we cannot see that there is anything to celebrate, if the cares, worries, distractions, and responsibilities of our common life have blinded us to the appropriateness and the possibility and necessity of celebration, heaven knows sex will not be playful. What's to celebrate? What's to be festive about? Why play?

And so, absentmindedly, casually, unreflectively, husband and wife make love. It is a private, profane encounter carried out with little sense of awe, reverence, or mystery. It unites them temporarily to each other, but it has no implications for their relationship with the rest of humankind, the cosmos, or the Primal Power. Technically competent they may be, physiologically and perhaps psychologically satisfied they may also be, but good God in heaven, playful they are not.

Sex is expansive. It increases—quite marginally, it is true—the amount of space our body occupies; it speeds up our physiological processes—heartbeat, blood flow, hormone secretion; it increases our physical energy and the madcap productivity of our imagination. It seems to fill us up until we are quite literally ready to burst. It also normally induces an emotional as well as physical "high." Our personalities expand at the same time. We feel bigger, more dynamic, more uninhibited. We are psychologically as well as physically excited, challenged, expanded.

When a man takes the body of his woman, when every inch of her flesh momentarily belongs to him, his sense of dignity, pride, masculinity, and power is elevated and transformed, or at least there is a strong strain in the encounter toward such a transformation. And when a woman is locked in an embrace with her man, when the last tatters of inhibition and restraint are put aside, her sense of elegance, beauty, fullness, strength, and power is dramatically enhanced, or at least the strain toward such enhancement is there. At such a time, pride in being a man or a woman and gratitude that one is a man or a woman become very strong. One can resist such pride and gratitude; one can deny it, one can repress it with guilt, prudery, disgust, or even hatred, but still the physiological and psychological forces are at work and draw both lovers toward pride and gratitude in each other as well as toward a raw and fundamental sense of pride in themselves.

Sex is an act of gratitude whether it is enjoyed or recognized. It is a celebration of the goodness in being a man or a woman, the goodness that is in being human with a capacity for sexual union. Sex is not merely communion; it is also Eucharist. It is an act of thanksgiving to the other, to the self, to whatever power there may be in the universe that has made this goodness possible.

One can certainly drain most of this communion and Eucharist dimension out of sex. Celebration can be denied, ignored, refused; but it is still there. It would be a mistake to underestimate the human capacity to deromanticize everything, to reduce even the most exciting events to the mundane and the commonplace. It would be even more a mistake to underestimate the capacity of the human creature to contend that such routinization is realism, wisdom, virtue, sophistication. In a desacralized, privatized world a contemporary human can get away with both routinization and its justification. Sex is ordinary; it is commonplace; it is unromantic, unsentimental, unexciting. There is in it nothing of communion, nothing of Eucharist, of ceremony, of celebration. Besides, there is a hard day to face tomorrow at the office, the club, the school. The feel of lips, neck, belly, thigh, buttocks has no meaning other than pleasurable sensation. One can touch a breast, stroke an arm, nibble on an ear, squeeze a rear end, run one's fingers through hair and still experience nothing more than localized sensation as a prelude to effective tension release. Celebration, communion, Eucharist? Don't be silly.

Okay, if that's the way you want it. But let it be clear that this sober realism, or puritanical or other quasi-religious variations of it, are entirely interpretations that the people involved choose to put on the event—a meaning they elect to assign to it for reasons of fear, infidelity, or shame that are all their own. There are other interpretations possible, perhaps harder to sustain but also infinitely more rewarding. Such interpretations do not deny that local sensation or tension release are involved, but they suggest that the immediate sensation is a revelation of something else, of love, of gratitude, fidelity, commitment, which may be focused indeed through the common life into the orgasmic embrace, but also out through the common life to place humankind, the cosmos, and whatever Power may have produced the cosmos. Playfulness simply cannot be sustained in a sexual relationship unless some one of these other interpretive schemes is applied to the lovemaking event. A woman's breast may simply be a sensitive gland that a man enjoys touching and a woman enjoys having touched. Or it may be a revelation of grace, love, and elegance in her, certainly, but also in the world of which she and her husband are a part. One can take one's interpretive position anywhere along the continuum between these two extremes, but the closer one gets to the second, the more likely sex is to be celebratory and hence playful. To unzip a zipper may be only that, or it may be the doorway to a place of excitement, delight, and pleasure. Which it is finally depends on how we choose to define it. And that definition and our acting on it will determine whether we are playmates or just mates.

The religious cop-out defines sex not as celebration, communion, and Eucharist, but for having children, rearing children, reducing concupiscence, keeping passions under control, and avoiding infidelity within the strictures of marriage. It is something best not talked about; it is animal, worldly, bodily; an embarrassment, disgrace, a regrettable necessity, or perhaps a necessary evil. (As St. Augustine suggests, it is at best a venial sin.) It is base, low, carried out in the same regions of the body where excretion takes place (*inter faces et urinam nascimur*, as the pagan poet so elegantly puts it). To use such words as "communion" or "Eucharist" concerning it is either romantic or idealistic or sacrilegious, quite possibly all three together. Life is a serious, responsible business; we must do all that we can to avoid committing mortal sin and thus losing our souls. It is hard enough to keep all the rules and all the commandments, to live up to all our responsibilities. There isn't much time for celebration. Sex is a burden, an obligation, a necessity. How could that possibly be both the cause and an occasion for celebration?

Even in this allegedly post-Freudian age of permissiveness the "religious" argument is pretty much in the form I have presented it here. Its underlying assumption is that religion must be life-suspicious if not life-denying. Humankind is not a creature to be trusted; his instincts, his passions, his hungers are dubious and dangerous. He must be controlled, restrained, disciplined, held in check. That is, after all, what religion is all about.

It may be what some religions are all about, but it is not what biblical religion is all about. As Professor Walter Bruggemann of Eden Theological Seminary notes in his book *In Man We Trust* (John Knox Press, 1972), "The wise in Israel characteristically appreciate life, love life, value it, and enjoy it. They appropriate the best learning, newest knowledge, and the most ingenious cultural achievements." Jesus told us that he came that we might have life and have it more abundantly. Even in the context of the New Testament that did not mean just life of the soul or life after death; it meant life for the human person, composite body and soul; life that would not end but life that would be more abundant now. Sex is part of life, the principle of life, the means by which life is continued. If Jesus came to bring us richer and more abundant life, then it is an inevitable consequence of his coming that our sex ought to be richer and more abundant. If it has not become so in the years that have elapsed since the appearance of Jesus, the fault is not in the brilliance or the clarity of his message but in our own fear and timidity and refusal to take him seriously, a refusal that consists essentially in not believing that when Jesus *said* "life" he *meant* life.

We do strain toward the transcendent, toward that which is beyond the here and now, beyond the confines of our segment of the time-space continuum. We do hunger for the absolute; we do seek that love which is eternally permanent. But we do not strain toward the absolute by running away from or denying or minimizing that love which exists to open up our personalities to a loving graciousness of the cosmos. A woman who thinks that she is obedient to the demands of absolute love when she restrains, restricts, and inhibits her passion for the man who shares her bed every night has a twisted notion at best of what love is and of what the graciousness is that Jesus revealed. A man whose relationship with his woman alternates between quick passion and silent shame may convince himself that this is a religious approach to the regrettably necessary filth of human sexuality, and he may do so in perfect good faith; but for all his good faith he thoroughly misunderstands that passionate God who revealed himself on Sinai, that Jesus who showed up at the marriage feast of Cana, and the religious implications of his wife's sexual attractiveness.

Both may argue that the life-suppressing or life-denying religious approach is what they were taught when they were growing up, and they may scapegoat "Catholic schools" for such teaching, implying that the schools deceived them and by this deceit dispensed them from modifying their attitudes in adult life. Heaven only knows that a lot of odd things were taught in Catholic schools, and that in its present manifestation Catholic Christianity is ill at ease with the life-affirming, life-endorsing themes of the Scripture—though in truth it is much less so than orthodox Protestantism. High-level Catholic theory does indeed assert that human nature is basically trustworthy, and that while man may be "wounded," he is not basically flawed, much less depraved. High-level theory even admits, grudgingly perhaps, that, despite the Augustinian tradition, the life-affirming, life-celebrating aspects of sexuality are good and wholesome and reflective and symbolic of God's passion for humankind. St. Augustine notwithstanding, the marriage rituals of the Catholic tradition down through the ages were simply unable to overlook the Cana dimension, that is to say, the celebratory aspect, of human sexual union.

The Protestant tradition, as Professor Bruggemann concedes, is much more suspicious of man, his life, his instincts, and his culture. But however strong the life-affirmation theories may have been in high-level Catholic theology, they filtered down erratically to the Sunday sermons, the catechisms, the textbooks, the marriage instructions. They grew badly confused in the endless controversy over what methods of family planning were appropriate—as though this were the only question of human sexuality on which the Catholic tradition could possibly shed any light. There were bits and pieces of teaching lying around from which many Catholics could, and some did, arrive at the correct conclusion that life is good and must be affirmed, that sex is admirable and must be celebrated. Such people enjoyed life and celebrated sex and paid rather little attention to what they read in the *Register* or the *Sunday Visitor* or heard from their parish priest on Sundays. Still, for most Catholic Christians it comes as a rude shock to be told that sex is a celebration and a eucharist to be celebrated. The logic is obvious enough and the conclusion may not be altogether implausible, yet it is a surprise to hear it.

A man may thoroughly enjoy squeezing his wife's buttocks as he presses her body against his, but to be told that this is not only not sinful but religiously admirable and possessed of a hint of divine graciousness is disconcerting. He had some difficulty in persuading himself that such delight is not dirty; now he is told that it is religious celebration. That may be the case, he admits, but no one ever told him that before, and it is a definition of religion that he finds startling. Still, unless he is incorrigibly puritanical, he may find himself more than a little intrigued by such a religion.

And the woman who has sufficiently overcome the sexual fears instilled in her by her mother and by the nuns who taught her in high school to be able to gently reach for her husband's penis when she awakens sexually aroused in the middle of the night may be somewhat surprised when she is informed that such action is not "base" but a form of eucharistic celebration, of ceremonial thanksgiving. Religion, as she remembers it, was a series of obligations dealing with things that one ought not to do and ought not to think. It was not a paradigm for festivity and celebration. Still a religion that comes down firmly on the side of more sex and better sex may not, after all, be a religion that she can write off as irrelevant.

But do either of these people really need a celebratory interpretive scheme to underwrite and reinforce their sexual life? The man does squeeze that soft and appealing area of his wife's anatomy, and she does reach for him in the middle of the night. Their biological urges, their human consequences and good taste, their affection for one another, their understanding of what it takes to keep a contemporary marriage alive and well have been sufficient for them to overcome their inhibitions, their fears, their guilts. They are capable of a fertile life, however hesitant and with whatever residues of past guilt feelings remain. Is a religion that tells them that these actions are Eucharist celebrations linked indeed in meaning and intention with the public celebration of the Eucharistic celebration that goes on in Church? What does that religion have to add to what is already occurring in their relationship?

There are, I think, three levels on which the question can be answered. A life-celebrating religious symbol system endorses and reinforces their sexual playfulness. It helps to sweep away the restraints, the fears, the inhibitions that may remain. Second, it encourages them to further exploration and growth together not only in their sex life but in all the dimensions and aspects of their common life together. Celebrations are self-regenerating. One good party deserves and demands another. One festive event leads us to want to plan another. Finally, and most important, a life-celebrating religion gives them the faith, the courage, and the hope they need to keep celebrating together when the going gets tough, and when the antilife forces, which are still powerfully at work in the cosmos, threaten to drain the vitality, trust, and hope out of their relationship. One need not even see this religious contribution taking place only in times of difficulty and crisis. It has been a bad day for both husband and wife. They have not exactly quarreled, but resentments, angers, frustrations, bitterness have built up. Her bottom still looks attractive and squeezable, but he is too angry to squeeze, and she is too angry to respond with anything but hostility. Yet if they believe in a passionately loving graciousness, whose goodness they celebrate in their common life together, each will lean toward graciousness to the other, and such a small difference can transform lives.

An explicit religious conviction about the graciousness of the Deity and sex as a celebration of that graciousness may be a resource that is not absolutely indispensable for a happy common life and a playful sexual relationship, but it doesn't hurt. When the chips are really down, people fall back on their ultimate interpretive scheme, and then, almost inevitably, the man and woman who believe explicitly and consciously in life-affirming graciousness can survive together the worst of times.

It is possible, then, to accept and live by a world view that affirms the goodness of life and of sexual union, and to believe that sex is celebration, communion, Eucharist. Under such circumstances, a religious context of sexual playfulness exists not merely in the marriage ceremony but in the daily lives of husband and wife. However, this celebration is still essentially private. It is not shared with others, and it is not part of religious ceremony outside of family life. Is there any way that sexual playfulness can be deprivatized and resacralized in the public domain? Can one share one's celebration with others while still keeping Church and community from "messing" in one's private life? All one can do at this stage of the development of thought is raise the question. Perhaps in centuries to come our inability to think out an answer to the question will be viewed by our descendants as bizarre. Still, the transition from objective playfulness to subjective playfulness in human sexuality is an awkward one. It is perhaps our misfortune to live right in the middle of the transition.

Two points can be made as footnotes to the discussion. First, the custom is growing for groups of married couples (usually three or four) to go away for a weekend together. Unlike Bob and Carol, Ted and Alice, everybody keeps to his own marriage bed. There is eating and drinking, swimming and dancing, perhaps even skiing and hiking. There is also a lot of sex; indeed the whole purpose of the weekend is that the husband and wife can get away from the home and children for a brief interlude of sexual abandonment. While each couple is having its own private orgy and comment about it may be restrained (or not), there is little doubt that the communal context is seen as enhancing the fun and games that go on in the individual bedrooms. Such elegant balance between privacy and communality, between group support and group orgy, may not be everybody's cup of tea, but it does indicate, I think, that some people are wrestling with the problem of keeping their sex lives private and still sharing the happiness and joy of their sexuality with friends without resorting to the barbarism and foolishness of spouse swapping.

There is also a tendency among some married people to ritualize or ceremonialize some of their lovemaking. Protocols of undressing, bathing, anointing are deliberately and consciously followed to enhance the sexual relationship and to guarantee that lovemaking is, at least on some occasions, not a hasty, casual, almost thoughtless encounter. Again, such ceremonials will not appeal to everyone, and will seem to some to be foolish and kinky. But such attempts to receremonialize intercourse indicate that despite the matter-of-fact mechanistic rationality of most of the sex manuals, many people have come to understand that sex and love are mysteries, and it is much more effective to celebrate mysteries than to try to understand them.

Throughout most of the course of human history men and women have realized (though usually not self-consciously) that sex was a mystery to be celebrated—in addition to all the other things it was. To contemporary human beings that notion—so obvious to their predecessors—seems strange, unreal, and dubious. When a man and woman begin to investigate the possibilities of sex as celebration, they feel awkward and uneasy and even guilty. For Catholics, in particular, there is irony as well as poignancy in this guilt. They had to overcome a lot of guilt to take sex out of the moralistic context in which it was seen as a remedy to concupiscence and something that was not sinful for married people so long as they were ready to produce numbers of children. With considerable effort (and not always with too much success) some Catholics are now able to think of sex as a normal, natural, healthy, expansive part of human life, and sexual playfulness as a desirable goal. Now they must overcome exactly the opposite guilt and resacralize sex. It is not merely a healthy, delightful, enjoyable part of life; it is also a revelation, a sacrament, the Eucharist, a participation in the basic life forces of the universe. As such, it must be uninhibitedly, wildly playful. For other Christians this transition has been spread over a couple of generations. But Catholics have been playing "catch-up" ball in recent decades and must cram many conflicting experiences into one generation. Whether one likes to have to shed two sets of guilt within one lifetime or not depends upon how resourceful or how playful one is or is willing to become. Some people may find it a splendid opportunity.

18

Playing is serious, but it is not the same as the "real world." The game of play is the game of make-believe, though it is not unreal. It has a different sort of reality than can be found in our mundane existence. We can be very serious about our game and still not confuse it with what might be appropriate concern for a sick child, with the consideration of a professional opportunity, or a threat to the peace of the world. We play the game to win, of course. A rout or a triumph can have effects on our mundane existence. Still, one invalidates the game by equating success or failure in life with winning or losing the game. When one does that, the barriers between play and the ordinary world break down, and the rules of the game have been violated.

Games also tend to be both fun and funny. One rarely sees a professional football player laugh at himself when he drops a forward pass. The Roumanian tennis star who seemed to think that the Forest Hills tennis championship was a splendid joke was considered a bit bizarre. For those of us whose living does not depend on how well we perform on the athletic field, it is somewhat easier to laugh at mistakes. A mighty swing and the golf ball dribbles off the tee, an agile leap on water skis over a wave only to be caught by the next and tumbled into the water, a smashing overhand shot and the ball is missed by a foot—these are the breaks of the game, and at our best moments we can laugh at them. The one who laughs too quickly is not deeply involved in the game, and the one who refuses to laugh at all has become so involved that he can no longer be playful. Both have failed to achieve the proper balance of serious engagement.

Professional athletics has become so major a business enterprise that such whimsical free spirits as Johnny "Blood" McNally are no longer permitted to frolic on the frozen turf of Green Bay, Wisconsin, on a late-autumn Sunday afternoon. A moderately bizarre character like Joe Kapp did not last very long; he was too erratic and unpredictable. And the incomparable Jim McMahon, the best quarterback in the history of the franchise, is always in trouble with Bear management. But professional athletes make up for the fact that business has squeezed the playfulness out of their game by their endless jokes and laughter (frequently lubricated by quantities of postgame, postseason booze). Don Meredith was unable to laugh at the Dallas Cowboys' annual loss to the Green Bay Packers while he was playing, but when he was a Monday-evening entertainer he managed to see the wry humor in what Green Bay had done to him every season.

Play, then, can be funny. There is a strain toward hilarity in the world of play. The strain can be resisted, the hilarity eliminated, but only at the risk of taking a great deal of the fun and pleasure out of the game. Sexual play is necessarily and inevitably funny. When a man and woman are not able to laugh with and at each other their relationship is certainly not playful. Laughter is both the cause and effect of playfulness in sex. It dispels strains, tensions, fears, and enables people to become playful.

That sex is funny does not need demonstration. It would appear that every culture the world has ever known has a tradition of "obscene" humor. Such humor is frequently crude, rude, and tasteless. It is also often cruel and exploitive, but it is also funny. Those who say that the dirty joke is "terrible" still manage to laugh at it. Neither theology nor social science has paid much attention to "obscene" humor. Theology has usually been content with denouncing the dirty joke as sinful, though conceding that among adults it is probably only a venial sin. Social science, when it pays any attention to the subject at all, usually does no more than footnote Freud's writing on wit and the unconscious. (One exception is the folklore collection *Rationale of the Dirty Joke: An Analysis of Sexual Humor* [G. Legman, Grove Press, 1968], a long, ponderous, and dreadfully dull encyclopedia of folk humor, which, for all its comprehensiveness, offers relatively little in the way of systematic interpretation.) One can't help but wonder what the reason is for such neglect. Everyone has heard dirty jokes; such a universal form of behavior must tell us something important about the human condition. Yet, it is swept under the rug. Surely in our permissive times the reason cannot be that people are afraid to discuss something as apparently trivial and base as obscene humor. That "permissiveness" of which we are so inordinately proud is dreadfully serious. There are many things we can show on a motion-picture screen that we never could before, but sexual humor doesn't seem to be one of them. Indeed, the old bedroom farces of the thirties and forties had a freedom to laugh about sex (without ever using the word) that our present heavy-handed cinematic protagonists of permissiveness do not seem to enjoy. One need only compare such dreadful and dour plays as *Hair* or *Oh! Calcutta* with the Restoration comedies to see the difference between serious sex and playful sex—and between exploitive fifth-rate art and creative talent. Puritanism persists in its illegitimate child, permissiveness. You can do just about anything you want with sex in contemporary America except laugh at it.

What is so funny about sex? The question must be answered on two levels. First, what are the aspects of human sexuality that trigger laughter? Secondly, why are we predisposed to respond with hilarity to sexual situations?

To begin with, the naked human body is funny. It may be radiantly beautiful, but it is also slightly ridiculous. A man or woman without clothes is caught in an embarrassing, absurd, awkward situation. We expect people to wear clothes, and when they don't it is a startling contrast. The dignity, the reserve, the aloofness, the coolness to which we pretend all slip away and we stand revealed in our alliance to the animal kingdom. All our fine pretensions to the abstract, theoretical, etherealized spirit dissolve in a cold blast of air on our goose-bumped bodies.

In our culture, where men are supposed to be far more interested in sex than women, part of the fun for a man in conquering a woman is to get her clothes off so that she stands revealed as being every bit as much a sexual being as he is. She may primly pretend not to be interested in sex, or not to be capable of sexual arousal, or to be able to suppress her sexual instincts; but get her clothes off and all that pretense is gone. Destroying pretense is, of course, a very laughter-provoking phenomenon in human culture. The drunk who pretends to be in complete control falls flat on his face and the crowd roars. The woman who pretends to be a sexless creature (at least relative to the superior sexuality of the man) loses her clothes and is revealed as thoroughly sexual after all. Her man laughs, although, if he is wise, only to himself.

In other cultures, where the woman is presumed to be the more highly sexed, it is very likely that the exact opposite phenomenon occurs. Even in our own culture a self-possessed woman with a sense of humor and a willingness to speak honestly about her reactions will admit that there is something mutually amusing in catching a man by surprise without his clothes on. His male dignity and his pretense at masculine superiority are snatched away from him, and he stands revealed as a creature who is as hesitant and uncertain about his sexual nature as is any woman. He reaches quickly for his clothes, his mask of male aloofness, but still he has been caught, found out, revealed; and the contrast between pretense and reality is laugh-provoking.

Laughter at the body of another can be cruel, particularly when it is a means of self-defense. But it need not be cruel. We can laugh at another body stripped of its clothes and pretenses with tenderness and affection. To the somber and the serious, it seems quite impossible to laugh at what one loves and finds beautiful, but one need only think of the laughter of parents at their children to realize how amusement, respect, affection, love can all be combined. The parent finds the child precious, important, beautiful, and also funny. One laughs at the little thing as he tries, oh so seriously and oh so awkwardly, to take his first steps across the room. He is beautiful, admirable, touching, and so funny; and these characteristics are so inextricably linked that we cannot separate them, and no one should bother to try.

So we love the body of our sexual partner and admire it and take pleasure in it and laugh at it because it is simultaneously beautiful, desirable, and funny. Any attempt to exclude one of these responses from the web of our reaction makes that reaction stunted and incomplete.

But if nakedness is funny, sexual arousal is even funnier (as much of the wit of "obscene" humor understands). We are curiously proud creatures, animal to be sure, but animals with a difference. We make elaborate pretenses at being superior to our fellow creatures (which we surely are) to such a degree that we are scarcely animal at all. We are self-disciplined, self-controlled, the master of our own emotions and our own destiny. We are the only animal that walks upright and even our simian relatives scurry along the ground on all fours very often. We can't do that anymore, and our upright stance is the symbol of our evolutionary superiority. We only need two limbs to move about, and we can thereby use the other two for implementing and executing the ingenious design our brains laid out for us. A superior creature indeed is humankind; his intellect controls and dominates everything he does. Other creatures are slaves to their instincts and their responses. Humankind creates his own meaning systems and then organizes the phenomena of life to fit these experiences. He has come down out of the trees, moved out of the forest, and walks through the fields and the streets of his cities on his hind legs. The Lord of Creation he unquestionably is.

(Actually, the comparison with animals is unfair to them: Their sexual couplings are quick and efficient and limited to certain times in a month or a year. Only the human animal is capable of and interested in sex almost all the time—a development in the evolutionary process designed to select for males and females who would remain together to rear their offspring. That which is specifically human in human sexuality [as distinct from the higher primates] is designed not for procreation but for bonding the couple together [quasi pair bonding because the binding energies can be resisted]. Hence the Catholic insistence that sex can always be designed for procreation seems to fly in the face of the natural law that the church purports to be defending.)

Lord of Creation humankind may be, but when he (or she) is sexually aroused much of that evolutionary superiority slips away. Unlike the reproductive interludes of other animals, those of human beings are fraught with meaning. They are self-conscious, self-reflective, self-defining acts. Still, they are fierce animal actions in which much of the self-control, self-discipline, and self-possession slips away. It is simply impossible to be in the full heat of sexual arousal and pretend that one is playing it cool and that one is immune to the power of fierce, nonrational forces. The contrast between the pose of complete self-possession, which humankind maintains most of

the time, and fierce animal desire, which dominates
the sexual encounter, is extremely funny—if not to
the aroused person himself then at least to those
who are watching him through the prism of a dirty
joke. Part of the fun of teasing one's sexual partner
certainly involves delight in making him ever so
slightly ludicrous. As one's partner becomes aroused
he is transformed from self-control and self-possession
to passionate hunger. That transformation is amusing to those who are sophisticated enough to enjoy
it. Sexual partners can do funny things to one another; they can tease, distract, take over the imagination, cause odd and peculiar transformations in the
shape, the rhythm, the color, and even smell of the
other body. In the process, the defenses, the dignity,
and the self-possession of the other slip away, and he
(or she) does indeed become rather like an amusing,
desirable, lovable child taking his first stroll from
chair to coffee table.

We lose our dignity in sexual encounters. While
lovemaking ought to be elegant, it can certainly
never be dignified or solemn the way other important events in our lives are. There is too much emotion, too much power, too much uncontrollable response, too much automatic and violent physical
response for us to maintain poses when we are making love. One of the reasons why lovemaking is in
most societies done privately is simply that so much
dignity is lost that we would be embarrassed to have
others see what wild animals we become in sexual
exchange.

Furthermore, most human activities are carried
on in an upright stance. Lovemaking usually occurs
in ungainly, awkward, uncomfortable, and slightly
ridiculous positions. The postures required to bring
together the sexual organs of a man and a woman

are very far from a beautifully choreographed ballet. The dignity of a creature who fancies himself mostly spirit and only inconsequentially animal is thrust away as he is gripped by the raw passions of his animal nature. Humans look ridiculous as they make love only because the contrast between their amorous thrashings and the dignity and self-control that mark their upright life is so dramatic. Sex is funny because it so devastatingly reminds us that we are both animal and spirit, and the pretense of the spirit to be free of and secure in its domination of the animal is at best a risky and tenuous position.

The richest, the most powerful, the most influential man in the world is reduced to the common denominator of our animal condition when he is sexually aroused, and the most aristocratic, refined, elegant woman is no different from any other woman when a man's body is united with hers. It is the capacity of human sexuality to bring everyone down to the same common denominator of our fundamental animal nature. There may be great pleasure in lying flat on one's back stark naked, one's legs spread apart, while someone else's body enters one's own; but there is no refinement, no daintiness, no self-possession at all in such a posture. There may also be great pleasure in mounting and plunging into the body that is now being possessed, but it is not pretty. They engage in their coupling in private partially because they know that what they are doing is in startling contrast to the way they normally behave and that others might find that contrast very funny.

When a man and woman make love to one another they also temporarily make fools out of themselves. They may suppress this fact and pretend that what they are doing is serious, sober, and dreadfully important. When this pretense is maintained in the face of almost overwhelming evidence to the contrary, the relationship between the man and woman offers the raw material for much of the high comedy the human race has produced. The intercourse interlude within such a relationship is responsible for almost all of our low comedy. Funny things happen when a man and woman make love to one another. They can pretend that it's not hilarious and thus protect their fragile egos, but such a pretense misses much of what goes on in the situation and absolutely precludes the possibility of sex's being playful.

One can laugh at oneself and one's sexual partner only in a context of a basically secure relationship. For laughter heals; it does not hurt. The little child trying to walk does not mind his parents' laughter, because he assumes that laughter and love are not inconsistent, and that laughter is simply another manifestation of love. If the husband and wife have developed a style in their marriage in which one is free to laugh because it is perceived as supportive and affectionate, then they will find it hard to control that laughter when they are having sex together. But if their relationship is heavy, somber, serious, responsible, then there is simply no way that they can begin to find anything amusing when the bedroom door is closed and their clothes are removed. When everything seems to be riding on the maximum amount of pleasure and success from this particular sexual encounter, the whole affair loses its humor entirely—which is, of course, a problem not only with serious marriages but with affairs that are too serious to be laughed at and hence too serious to be playful.

A man and woman who are close to one another develop a whole private agenda of shared jokes, frequently shared in a code that is only understood by the two of them. A shared joke becomes even funnier if it is a secret one. This secret agenda of shared laughter may include hilarious experiences in the whole of their common life, including those that occurred in bed. No couple's agenda of shared wit will be just like any other couple's; no one can prescribe for others what they will find funny (though heaven knows some sex manuals try). Private jokes are private jokes; by definition they can be imposed by no one else.

One couple, for example, goes into uncontrollable laughter whenever someone else uses the word "plunger." Their friends didn't exactly understand what they were laughing at, and thought it best not to ask. However, one night after the "creature" had flowed liberally, the couple told their friends why that word was so funny. For reasons that they couldn't explain the two of them found the "plopping" sound made when the husband's sweat-soaked body pulled off the wife's breasts, to which he had become "glued" during lovemaking, to be an incredibly funny phenomenon. It sounded so much like the noise of a plunger cleaning a drain that they began to call this aspect of their lovemaking "the plunger effect." It invariably brought their sex exchange to an end in peals of laughter.

Others might not even notice such an experience, might not think it particularly funny, and certainly would not look forward to it as a pleasant bit of frosting on the cake. But what others might think makes no difference. For this particular couple this quite ordinary and trivial sound has become a shared joke, a shared delight, and a pleasant bit of their comic game, a game that was *theirs* and no one else's.

We share jokes only with our friends. Indeed, we normally tell dirty jokes only to those we are sure will let us get away with it. Hence we can appreciate the humor, the wit, the incongruity, the foolishness of our sexuality only when it is shared with a close friend. Casual, transient sex simply cannot be funny, because the background of common experience, the preexisting agenda of shared jokes into which the laughter of this particular interlude can be fit, is not there. Transient sex is necessarily serious. We are afraid of laughter because we assume, usually correctly, that it will be interpreted as hurting rather than healing laughter. Only after a sustained relationship has been built can we be sure that our partner is laughing with us and not at us.

At a deeper level, laughter serves to reduce aggression and reduce fear. Psychiatrists agree that laughter is a form of aggression, but it need not hurt nor be intended to hurt. It communicates something that is important and demanding but with the barb removed or blunted. If we are angry at someone else we can get rid of it by losing our temper or by diverting it into laughter, which simultaneously releases the angry energies and enriches and enhances the relationship. Laughter is a safety valve that enables us to get a perspective on our own aggressive emotions and share them with the other in a way he can accept and deal with. Two people who live together in the oppressive intimacy of a sustained sexual union either will develop a way of communicating much of their aggressions through the soft language of laughter, or they will repress the aggression, or they will tear one another apart. Laughter is obviously the most attractive of the three alternatives.

But above all, laughter dispels fear. It is, as Peter Berger points out in his *A Rumor of Angels*, a blunt assertion from humankind that it is not afraid even of death. All laughter is a laughing at death, according to Berger, and at those fears and anxieties that are ultimately rooted in death.

Sex is a scary business, which explains why so many of the psychological disturbances that afflict humankind are sexual either in their origins or in their manifestations or both. In sex we put ourselves on the line both physically and psychologically in a way we do in practically no other kind of activity. (Public speaking is another and related form of self-exposure that evokes related forms of terror and delight.) The confident, supreme, certain lover is a faker, who cannot admit to himself or anyone else that he shares the common lot of humankind, that he too is afraid of sex. The theologian John Dunne in his book *Time and Myth* (Doubleday, 1973) suggests that fear of sexuality is linked to our primal fear of death: "Sexuality is not only fascinating but dreadful, it seems, for it is experienced as a terrible purpose at work in one's life, a purpose that is not personal but somehow impersonal in its themes, a purpose that looks to the species rather than the individual, to the reproduction of one's kind rather than to one's own personal development. If we were to ask, 'Why do we fear our sexuality?' we would undoubtedly be told that we fear it because we have been taught to fear it, because we have learned to see it as fraught with moral danger. In reality, though, the fear seems to go well beyond merely learned fears. It is like the fear of death. We could be told also that we have been taught to fear death, that we fear it because we have learned to fear it. Yet death seems in fact to be inherently fearful. Actually, we fear both our sexuality and our mortality for the same reason, it seems, because they are forces within us that drive beyond all personal goals, that threaten our personal existence by leading beyond it."

If Dunne is right, and it seems to me that he is, then the naive notion, so popular in our time, that we can stop being afraid of sex if we can get rid of the silly and ignorant fears we acquired from our family, our schools, our churches is a foolish self-deception. The goal of "sex without fear" is a false one, and energies wasted on it are invested in self-deception. It would be much better to deal with sexual fear by not denying it or writing it off as a residue of an unenlightened past, but by respecting it, understanding it, coping with it, and transcending it.

A man and woman locked in a sustained relationship with each other are crazy if they do not acknowledge that there is fear in that relationship. The other is so close, knows one so well, and has so much power and influence over one. Ridicule, betrayal, infidelity can break a heart, and the other has the power to use them if he (or she) chooses. There is pleasure in being afraid of that other and in acknowledging it. Indeed, it may be possible to engage in playfulness only when that fear is out in the open and can be laughed at together.

Laughter in sex, then, is a response to fear, and the ultimate origins of sexual humor can be found, I suspect, in our fear of the awesome power of sex, a power, as Father Dunne points out, that draws our life out beyond ourself. We laugh at death and we laugh at sex because if we don't laugh at them they may well overwhelm us. We laugh also because of the stubborn conviction, irresistibly present in the depths of our personalities, that in the long run we will have the last laugh at the terrors of death and at the terrors of sex. They both may draw us out beyond our own personal existence, and when we get out there we stubbornly believe, at least part of the time, that what we feared turns out not to be fearsome at all.

So lovers laugh together at themselves and at one another because they are afraid of the power of their sexuality, because they are afraid of one another, but also because they are convinced that they can transcend the fear and find out that their sexuality and their sexual fears are even more delightful than they are terrifying. That delight conquers terror is a basic and fundamental human religious hope. It is a hope, incidentally, that Jesus came into the world to confirm. The revelation of God's love as grounds for hope stands as solid reinforcement for the uncontrollable laughter of true lovers who are swept away by the delights they experience in playing with one another.

But if laughter is a response to fear—indeed, the only effective response—it is also severely inhibited by fear. We are afraid to laugh. Our sexuality and our sexual union are serious and important matters. Much of our life happiness will depend upon them; they are not matters to be taken lightly. Therefore it seems inappropriate, almost blasphemous, to laugh. Sex is horrifying, shameful, vile, base, depraved on the one hand; but on the other, sexual orgasm is absolutely indispensable for self-fulfillment and to prove our masculinity or our femininity and to keep a marriage together. To the puritan and the hedonist, sex is surely not a laughing matter.

Sex without humor becomes cruel. For either we release our aggressions and dispel our fears with laughter or we protect ourselves from what the other may do to us. Cruelty is one of the best forms of self-protection that the twisted human psyche has ever produced. It is hard not to laugh at the awkward, ungainly, undignified interlude of sexual encounter, but we can repress it; we can make the event somber, serious, and most people manage to do it most of the time. Fear doesn't go away, of course, but it does get repressed, and then seeps out in vengeful, destructive, and punitive disguises. Instead of sex being too important to laugh at, it is too important not to laugh at.

Life is a mixture of comedy and tragedy. We deny the existence of one or the other only at the risk of deceiving ourselves. The basic question is not whether we can dispense with either comedy or tragedy but whether comedy might just not possibly be ever-so-slightly more powerful than tragedy. Sex, the fundamental life-giving power, reflects the ambiguity of life. It is both terror and delight. If we believe that delight is ever-so-slightly more important than the terror, then we are free to laugh. But, paradoxically, in our freedom to laugh we discover that the power of delight exorcises terror. The husband and wife who share the crude little joke about "the plunger effect" may have many problems in their relationship. It is unlikely that fear has been completely eliminated from their sexual life (it can never happen in this world), but they do have a joke they share. When anger, hatred, or fear threatens to disrupt the playfulness of their union, there is always the joke to help dispel these enemies. If their intelli-

gence is sophisticated they will not deny the fear
involved in their sex, for if sex is not something
important and powerful enough to be afraid of, then
it is likely to be uninteresting and dull. But their
joke and the context of humor and play that surrounds it will help keep fear at bay. Whether their
joke is a reflection of a great Cosmic Joke in which
life successfully puts down death remains to be seen.
It is not necessary that they see their "plunger effect" as a reflection of the Cosmic Joke, but it won't
hurt them if they do.

19

From one perspective playful sexuality seems to be the easiest thing in the world. Playfulness is built into the psychological and physiological dynamics of the situation. It is hard for sex not to be festive, fantastic, humorous. A man and woman should develop patterns of playing together that are as easy and as natural as an apple falling off a tree. But in fact we know that relatively few couples do indeed develop such patterns of playfulness. Many will even argue that playfulness is a romantic, sentimental, idealistic illusion. Temptations against playfulness must be strong indeed if they are able to overcome what seems to be an almost natural propensity.

Let us take several examples of relatively minor sexual playfulness.

It is a summer afternoon. The husband is drowsing on the couch; the children are outside playing. The wife comes up to the couch, runs her fingers through his hair, and as he awakens from his nap, she begins to gently kiss him—his eyes, nose, ears, forehead, lips, chin. The kisses are at first bare touches, but the strength and power of them build up. She concludes with an extremely passionate, lingering, inviting, overwhelmingly suggestive kiss on his lips. At that point she leaves quickly for the yard, leaving him very much awake.

The man comes home from work just as his wife is getting out of the shower. He takes the towel from her hands and begins to dry her off. She protests at first that she must get dinner ready. But then, as he briskly and competently moves the towel over her body, she accepts his ministrations docilely, her eyes growing wider with pleasure and anticipation. He pats her derriere and tells her to get on with the business of dinner.

The husband is on the telephone for what is a long and important call. His wife comes up behind him, puts her arms around him, and squeezes hard. She then begins to gently nibble on the back of his neck, distracting him from his phone call. He doesn't seem to mind enough to push her away, but just as the call is coming to an end she leaves him to busy herself with something else.

Husband and wife are in the back of a car going somewhere with friends. The husband's hand creeps under her skirt and moves slowly up her thigh. She makes a face and tries, not too convincingly, to push him away. His hand continues its exploration of the sensitive areas, and when they arrive at the party his wife has many other things on her mind.

The two of them are in the front seat of their own car in stop-and-go traffic. The husband's driving is frustrated and impatient. His wife's hand, which was resting on his arm, seeks another area of his

body, and the husband finds his waiting for the
traffic to move substantially more easy to bear.

Guests are due in five minutes. The wife is putting on finishing touches in front of the mirror. The
husband walks by and suddenly finds his wife's back
extremely attractive. He deftly unhooks her bra,
squeezes her breasts against her body, covers her
back with kisses, and murmurs passionately what a
beautiful woman she is. The interlude lasts but a
minute; the doorbell rings, and the guests begin to
arrive.

A number of things are to be noted about all of
these incidents. They are utterly trivial and commonplace. They are minor in the sense that they
require little activity and not much in the way of
immediate response. They are gratuitous in that they
are easy to do, make almost no demands on time,
and run no risk of shocking children. (Would children be shocked to find their mother kissing their
father? One hopes not!) They interfere not in the
least with serious obligations and responsibilities.
They are supportive, euphoric, quite unnecessary,
spontaneous, simple, easy. In a way it is almost
hard not to do them. Such actions, or at least those
like them, are simply manifestations of spontaneous,
natural, impulsive propensities of sexually healthy
men and women living in close proximity to each
other. A squeeze, a touch, a kiss, a caress, a nibble, a
period of exploration—there are few things in life
that can be done more cheaply or easily. They are
quintessentially playful.

They are jokes, tricks, games, teases. They are
exercises in fantasy and minor tidbits of festivity. In
such situations the inclination to indulge in such
playfulness is very strong. It is what virtually every-

one would like to do in such circumstances, and yet what very few manage to do.

The opportunities are there; the payoff is evident; the procedure is clear; and still nothing happens. Are there sexual hang-ups? Probably. But the real problem goes deeper than sexuality. If a man and woman, pushed together in the intimacy of their common life, cannot or do not respond the way their spontaneous impulses incline them, the flaw in their personalities and their relationship is human rather than only sexual.

Before they came together they fantasized a life that would be filled with certain spontaneous exchanges of affection, enticement, and encouragement. But they somehow never got started, or, perhaps, they have long since stopped what began so tentatively and never developed. In their daydream relationship they may act like tender, playful lovers; but in the real world they share together, playfulness and affection are restrained, inhibited, and repressed. If they are asked why, they might respond that other things are more important than sex in their life together, or that they have so many commitments, responsibilities, or distractions, or that sex just isn't so important as it used to be, or that we could hardly expect them to act like children or adolescents.

All of these answers may be true. The adjustment they have worked out together may be a satisfactory one, on the whole, for both of them. No one can seize all the opportunities in life, and if two people choose to focus on other opportunities that they think are incompatible with sexual playfulness, then that is their decision. But I must raise the question whether their whole existence might not be constrained, cautious, conservative, careful, and that a constricted sexuality is merely the reflection of a

constricted adjustment to life. May not their fundamental lifestyle be a "no"? No to possibility, no to
risk, no to delight, no to reward. May they not have
turned away from the opportunity of playfulness
because their fundamental response to everything in
life is a turning away from opportunity?

I must admit that my three decades of working
with young people have made me very melancholy
about humankind in its present state of development. The lives of most of the young people I watched
grow up are lives of easy opportunities needlessly
lost. Their marriages and sexual relationships are
just the most acute and obvious symbol of the "no"
that is said to all the opportunities of their lives. They
are cautious, conservative, cynical not at thirty-five or
forty but already at twenty-five, and some are that
way at seventeen and eighteen. The great outburst of
student activism in the sixties (itself a badly flawed
and extremely deceptive phenomenon) blinded us to
the fact that the young of today are even more
cautious and conservative than their Depression-born
parents. I do not know how one goes about preparing
people to seize easy opportunities, particularly when
the basic system that filtered to them through their
parents and was reinforced by their teachers and
clergy led them to believe that life is dangerous,
punitive, repressive, and that the wise person takes
no risks at all. Poets, novelists, political leaders,
mystics, scholars, saints have all gone down the
drain of cynicism and caution. Who in their right
mind would expect such people to be playful lovers?

Their lives are filled with fear, anger, shame,
dullness, cowardice, routine, monotony. They protect
themselves from risk and punish those closest to
them because they dared to threaten the thick armor

plating of self-sufficiency, which they use to protect their frail, frightened egos.

Married couples pile up vast quantities of anger and hatred toward one another in a life together. Not infrequently it becomes more important to punish, to inflict pain on the other, than to do anything else in life. It is all done implicitly, subtly, indirectly—though when the two have had enough to drink at a party, it is likely that the pain will burst out into the open. One resists the impulse to play with the other because the other might like the experience, and to deprive him or her of such pleasure is just about the only really meaningful reward left in life.

The wife passes by the husband dozing on the couch and the thought of teasing him with her kisses rises spontaneously in her imagination, but, "Kiss the son of a bitch? He should be out mowing the lawn."

The husband glances into the mirror and sees his wife combing her hair. The impulse to squeeze her and to tell her how yummy she looks is very strong, but he doesn't like the guests she invited and is not about to reward or encourage her before a party that is bound to be a drag. Punishment in both cases is more important than pleasure.

This may not be exactly the totality of the human condition, but unfortunately it is the way a very considerable number of people freely choose to live. It is easier to say "no" than to say "yes" to life. Once you affirm life, you deprive yourself of a very considerable capacity to inflict pain and suffering on those you hate (or love).

Father Dunne, in *Time and Myth*, notes that we miss the whole point of James Joyce's *Ulysses* if we think it is merely about adultery in Dublin. For Ulysses has returned to Penelope, and we have here not merely twentieth-century Dublin but a classical, mythological theme and a fundamental human existential question. Does one say "yes" or "no" to the possibilities of life? At the mythological level the two lovers are saying "yes."

> I asked him with my eyes to ask again yes and then he asked me would I say yes to say yes my mountain flower and first I put my arms around him yes and drew him down to me so he could feel my breasts all perfume yes and his heart was going like mad and yes I said yes I will Yes.

Think what we will about Joyce and the characters who inhabited Dublin at the beginning of the century, the question of "yes" or "no" is not only sexual; it is the most basic and fundamental human and religious question that can be asked. Does one want to live fully or cautiously? Does one wish to be open or constricted, risk-taking or cynical? Playful people have playful sex, and their sexual playfulness reinforces and strengthens their playfulness as people. We become playful people only when we say "yes" to the opportunities that the Spirit of Life, with implacable insistence, offers us every day. For most people, the sexual partner to whom they are committed in a sustained relationship is the biggest single opportunity they will ever receive. It is the decisive opportunity, and whether they say "yes" or "no" will shape everything else that happens in their lives. If they say "no" they might just as well subscribe to *Playboy* or *Playgirl* because that is as close to playful sex as they will ever get.

20

I am surprised by the durability of puritanism. It may be that I am more a victim of the folklore about permissiveness and sexual revolution and hedonism than I had thought. I wrote the previous essay, *Sexual Intimacy*, more or less by accident in response to a request for a pamphlet. After a couple of decades of pre-Cana and Cana conferences and the second Vatican Council, the confusion of Freudian psychology, and the relaxation of many of the more rigid sexual taboos of years gone by, I would have thought that puritanism would be in full retreat. One could write, it seemed to me, a very frank essay about human sexuality as an occasion for religious reflection on the meaning of sexuality. One need no longer be reticent about discussing the human body and its functions, about referring to sexual organs by their proper names, reflecting on the function of nudity and clothing on eroticism, and the development of a personal eroticism without having to fear the reaction. It turned out, however, that I had underestimated the strength of puritanism.

The puritanical response to *Sexual Intimacy* represented much less than the majority of those who wrote, but what astonished me about my puritanical correspondents was not that they disagreed with my approach but the vile, angry, hate-filled style of their disagreement. The puritan writers did not even bother to try to understand what was being said. The context of a chapter or of the whole book was irrelevant. Certain words had been mentioned, certain images had been suggested, certain practices described, and that was enough to drive some letter writers to paroxysms of fierce anger.

As the man says, they do protest too much. They reveal more of their own unconscious and their own fantasy life than they could possibly imagine.

I was naive, of course. Puritanism is a remarkably strong element in human culture, and it will take a good deal more than a few half-baked and shallow "sexual revolutions" to sweep it aside. One cannot argue with a puritan, and I shall attempt to do no more of it in this essay than I did in its predecessor. But the real problem is the tendency toward puritanism that exists in all of us; it is a dimension of practically all human beings that antedates Christianity. It managed to grip the early Christian religion in its clammy paws and took on Christian colors, the fakery and gaudiness of which have only recently become obvious to a few Christians. Puritanism is the ultimate sexual temptation, and in a way it is the ultimate human temptation. It is a decisive "no" to human sexuality, a decisive "no" to human goodness, a decisive "no" to the Gracious Vitality of the universe.

Puritanism is fundamentally a fear of sexuality. The puritan quite correctly notes that sex is dangerous simply because it cannot always be dominated by human rationality; it breaks out in wild, passionate, uncontrolled feelings and actions. It threatens chaos, so it must be evil, and the less we have to do with it the better off we will be. The Platonists, the Manichees, the Gnostics, all the ancient spiritualist heresies believed that man was Spirit, that the body imprisoned man, and that human sexuality, so obviously and painfully a function of the body, was the worst of the demons that bound and caged the human Spirit. More primitive people were superstitious in their fears of sexuality. They knew what sexual arousal could do to a warrior; it could deprive him of his will to fight. They knew that a sexually aroused woman was insatiable. They knew that sexuality kept the tribe in existence, but they also recognized that it could unleash forces that could tear the tribe asunder. The forces of sexuality had to be disciplined, controlled, restrained; and so an elaborate system of taboos was set up to keep this fearsome power under control. The Israelite religion was more relaxed on the subject of sexuality than either the nature religions or the Near Eastern heresies that were Platonic in inspiration. Still the Hebrews did hedge sexuality in with an elaborate set of rituals and stipulations. They remembered the fertility goddesses their ancestors had fought in the hill shrines of Palestine, and while now fertility was seen as the dutiful servant of Yahweh, the Israelites were not about to take chances.

The recognition of human weakness, which is strong in St. Paul, stronger still in St. Augustine, and very strong indeed in the Lutheran and classical reformers, provided a perfect opening for puritanism to creep in and almost take possession of Christianity. For more than a millennium and a half few if any Christian theologians had much of a kind word to say about sexuality—despite the sexual imagery that can be found in many different places in the Scripture (Jeremiah, Ezekial, Hosea in the Old Testament and the Gospels and Epistles in the New). The puritans have had things all their own way in the theory of human sexuality (save in the marriage rituals and ceremonials). Indeed, in the minds of many Christians, and particularly Catholic Christians, the puritan style is indistinguishable from the Christian style. Sex is base, vile, dirty, shameful; it ought not to be discussed. It is basically a means for satisfying concupiscence and reproducing the human race.

Christianity is now in the process (under substantial prodding from the Freudians) of exorcising puritanism from the Christian tradition. It will not be an easy task. Puritanism survived as long as it has because it turns out to be a useful shield under which fear can hide.

Sex is demonic, make no mistake about it. It does unleash fierce and not altogether controllable powers in the human personality. It is ecstatic; it snatches human beings out of their ordinary modes of existence. Anything that is ecstatic and demonic must be approached with some caution and reserve. Fear of human sexuality seems to be built into the human condition, and it is a good thing to be afraid of it. The naive optimist who thinks that sexuality is something nice, neat, and natural, making no problems for anybody once they have shed all their "hang-ups," is kidding himself. There is a dark side to sex as well as a bright side, a destructive dimension as well as a constructive one. The wise person respects the demonic and the ecstatic elements of his sexuality. They can get him into trouble. They can make him do things that are hurtful to both him and others. Like all creative powers sexuality must be treated with some caution, some restraint and care. Such a viewpoint—offensive perhaps to encounter-group hedonism—is sensible, discreet, wise.

But it doesn't go far enough for the puritan. It is not merely enough for him to caution about sex, one must also pronounce a condemnation of it. It is not enough to say that nothing excuses man from an exercise of rationality. Sex is not only nonrational, it is irrational. The rational man will have as little to do with it as possible.

One does not go nearly as far as the puritan wants when one says that sex is demonic; it must also be added that it is diabolic. One does not satisfy the puritan when one says that sex is ecstatic; it must also be said that it is evil. The puritan does not want to hear that we should have a healthy respect for the power of sexuality to get us into trouble. What he wants to hear is a simple statement that sex will always get us into trouble. When he is told that sexuality shapes human dignity because it reasserts the fundamental animal component of our personality, he is delighted. Animality is base, low, and wrong. When we act "like animals" we stop being human, which is, of course, evil. When we contend that sexuality is a complex, intricate problem that no one ever understands perfectly, he agrees with us and adds that the best way to cope with the problem is to have as little to do with it as possible.

The puritan's response to human sexuality is that if you wish to avoid the danger, the difficulty, and the complexity of human sexuality, you condemn it and then try to stop sexual activity. It would be nice, the puritan admits, if people could be trusted with their animality, their sexuality, their passions; but obviously you can't trust them. So the best thing to do is to tell them that their passions are bad and that they should enjoy them as little as possible. That way we will protect people from the difficulty of making decisions, from the awesome responsibility of balancing passion and rationality. Life, the puritan argues, may not be quite as much fun if you accept his perspective, but it's a lot safer.

The puritan won't admit it, but sexuality, like all the other nonrational forces that sweep through the universe and inundate the human personality, is a trap, a temptation, a trick that an arbitrary, cantankerous, suspicious God is playing on humankind to see if we are smart and brave and tough enough to resist the temptation and avoid the dangers into which we are being tricked.

It is an interesting view of God, a not uncommon one in Christian and Catholic circles (the old Irish monsignor image of God). It has relatively little to do with the Yahweh of Sinai or the Jesus of Cana, but if the puritans are right and God is of the sort they say he is instead of the sort Jesus says he is, then we had better be pretty damn careful. For the Holy Spirit is not a benign trickster then, a playful imp, a poltergeist, a laughing spirit, a leprechaun; she is a mean, vindictive character who is abroad in the cosmos to trip us up, make fools of us, and send us off to hell if she possibly can. In the puritan world view, the Holy Spirit seems quite indistinguishable from Satan. Hence it is understandable that that which is demonic (and of the Spirit) must also be seen as diabolic.

Puritanism comes to terms with the fearfulness of the cosmos of life and of sexuality by running from it. One either laughs or runs; the puritan says: "Run while you can. Run for your life!"

Puritanism is a religious world view. It doesn't happen to be a Christian world view, but it is religious; and within its own framework it is a consistent, serious, and devout religion. But it also turns out to be a very useful religion for underwriting no-saying. Indeed it turns "no" into an act of highest virtue. It is a defense against the attractiveness of others, a defense against the outgoing dimensions of our own personality. It is a defense against the consuming demand to come forth that we hear from within ourselves and from some other or Other, who seems to be calling to us from Out There. Puritanism tells us that our safe, cynical, life-denying propensities, which we would like to indulge anyhow, represent the highest of human virtues. Do you want to be good? Fine. Deny life, deny love, deny risk, deny pleasure, deny delight. Just as the hedonist says, "Enjoy, enjoy," and the guilt-ridden liberal says, "Expiate, expiate," the puritan says, "Deny, deny."

Puritanism has another use. It's a marvelous way of hating and punishing other human beings under the guise of virtue. We obtain strong ego reinforcement by identifying with the cause of righteousness and virtue and by being shocked and outraged by all the immorality that swirls around. There is a curious lack of consistency and pattern in this sense of outrage. A pinup picture and a full-blown Rubens, a dirty joke and a scanty swimming

suit, *Ulysses* and hard-core pornography, young people kissing in a car and rape—all merit equally
violent outrage from the puritan. By donning the
mantle of goodness and virtue the puritan can be as
nasty, as vicious, as vindictive, and as punitive as he
wants. Everything he does, he argues, is done to
protect virtue and morality.

The puritan is likely to be married, and as such
he will occasionally "have sex." It is not important
in his marriage, he will insist. He and his spouse love
each other; they share many things in common, of
which sex is only a relatively minor part. The principal joy in his marriage is his children, and he must
do all he can to protect the morals of his children
from corruption. (So off to the neighborhood drug-
store to censor the magazine rack.) Sex is a burden
that one must live with, but it ought not to be
discussed or mentioned and only enjoyed in the
strictest moderation. The very idea that sex should
be playful strikes him as blasphemous. Or, as one
puritan commented to me, "The Church was much
better in the past when we never heard a thing about
sex."

But for the puritan it is not enough that he drain
the enjoyment out of his own sexuality; it is necessary for others to deny the enjoyment of theirs.
Playfulness is not something to be renounced because of one's own taste; it is something to be de-
nounced in others as fundamentally immoral and
irresponsible. Horror, shock, dismay, anger—these are
the stock-in-trade of the puritan when he hears the
faintest suggestion that for other people sex might
be fun.

And if the puritan happens to be married to
someone less puritanical, then the other is in deep
trouble. The slightest hint that sexual pleasure and

playfulness might be expanded is greeted with absolute horror and outraged harshness. "Don't you even think of anything like that ever again!" This is the puritan's response to the most harmless sexual innovation. It's bad enough for one to "have sex," but to make it frivolous or foolish or festive or fantastic is simply inviting the heavens to call down their outraged puritanical punishments on people who could be so vile.

What can one do with a puritan? Not much, I fear. The puritan has made his religion so much a part of his world view and his personality that you can neither argue with him nor seduce him out of it. The person who is a self-conscious, principled puritan is incorrigible. Others may be reluctant puritans, trapped by their childhood experiences and their education into puritan attitudes and habits that they don't like and from which their intelligence tells them they ought to escape. Such reluctant puritans are enough to try the patience of a saint, and those of us who have to deal with them often have an impulse to shake them until they come to their senses. Gentleness, kindness, patience, persistence—and not infrequently psychotherapy—may help to liberate them. When there is a marriage between two such reluctant puritans (and in contemporary Catholicism, alas, such matches are all too frequent), one is presented with a very difficult relationship indeed. The prognosis must certainly be guarded; still, as the Scripture says, with God all things are possible. (And be it noted that in this context the Scripture is talking about getting a camel through the eye of a needle.)

I am not sure that a thoroughgoing, convinced puritan is really capable of marriage. The canon lawyers will probably have to figure this out (and they may get to it in another hundred years or so), but whether someone who believes in fundamental principles as well as daily practice that sexuality is evil can really enter a contract for a sustained sexual union seems to me to be quite dubious. The puritan who will not give up his puritanism or will not even try to give it up is more than a little mad, I think. And given what we have come to believe marriage is, his capacity for marriage must be considered minimal indeed.

But the convinced puritans are not as much a problem as the partial, reluctant puritanical aspects of our own personalities that still affect us. The puritan strain in us is such a marvelous excuse; it justifies, rationalizes, and reinforces no-saying. It underwrites our little acts of meanness and vindictiveness. It makes us feel guilty about our hesitant attempts to be playful, and urges us to quit when these attempts are not immediately successful. It strengthens our shame, our fear, our anxieties, our self-loathing, our disgust. It argues vigorously about our responsibilities, our commitments, about the seriousness of life. It shrugs its shoulders and says, "Well, after all, sex isn't everything." (Although no one ever claimed that it was.)

Puritanism will persist as long as fear of sex persists. It has been dealt a decisive blow by contemporary psychology and some of the more recent theological reflection on that psychology. Human history is not all circle; progress does occur, and we have made progress against puritanism. It would have been impossible even ten years ago for someone within Catholic Christianity to write a book of theological reflections on sexual playfulness. (It's still a bit risky, but by and large safe.) It would be foolish to think that puritanism will release its clammy grip on Christianity without a fight. It may take several more generations before liberation from puritanism will have been substantially accomplished. In the meantime we will have to put up with a good deal of nonsense about sexual revolutions, sexual permissiveness, and the new sexuality. Much of this nonsense, incidentally, is in reality cryptopuritanism, attempting to impose a whole new set of sexual obligations to replace the old. The hedonist's injunction, "Enjoy, enjoy," is as absolutely moralistic as the puritan's "Deny, deny."

The defeat of puritanism will not mean, as such half-witted utopian visions as *The Harrod Experiment* would have us believe, that the human race can enjoy sex without fear. For sex without fear would be sex without passion and that would be no sex at all. The goal is rather more modest and more realistic: sex without unreasonable or inappropriate fear, sex that is enjoyable, playful, rewarding, festive, fantastic, and funny, and sex that at the same time recognizes its own demonic and ecstatic dimensions. It is precisely that which gives sex its mystery, its depth, its power, and its strength that also makes it frightening. Between the hedonism that sees only delight and the puritanism that sees only terror there ought to be a middle path that sees both terror and delight, with delight strong enough to laugh at terror and thereby make even it delightful. You won't find that middle course through Harrod experiments or sexual communes or wife swapping. You will only get it through slow, patient development of skills, insights, and understanding in the sexual game. And that, to repeat once again the basic theme of this volume, is a lifelong task.

21

Love is play; play is love. Both defy death.

Just as children only play with those who are friends, so sexual partners only play with those they love. Love precedes play and follows it. It makes possible the atmosphere of trust, confidence, of festivity, fantasy, and wit that is essential for play to begin. Play, in turn, enhances all these characteristics in a common life together. You can, it would seem, love someone intensely and not be playful. Parents can have a deep and abiding love for a child and still resist all inclinations to play with that child. In principle, I suppose that such a relationship between parent and child is not wrong, but not to play with a child when the spontaneous impulses of both the adult and childish natures would lead you to that playfulness is, to say the least, rather strange. Your relationship with the child may still be a good one, but there is something missing.

Similarly, it is possible to have a good relationship with a spouse without the lightness, the laughter, the teasing, the jokes, the surprises that constitute play. Certainly there are many married people with good relationships whose sexual lives are serious, restrained, utterly devoid of playfulness. Again, there is nothing "wrong" with such marriages, but something is missing.

Playfulness reinforces love, but love does not necessarily generate playfulness, although there is a spontaneous impulse in that direction once love is permitted freedom. It is the thought of death, explicit or implicit, that inhibits love and restrains playfulness.

Father Ladislaus Boros notes (in *Hidden God*, Seabury Press, 1973) that to love means to say, "You will not die."

> Love confers immortality upon the beloved human being....It cannot be that you will leave me forever. It cannot be that you are given over to eternal destruction. It cannot be that there can be never again the possibility of your developing into that which I saw in moments of inner vision....Faith in the immortality of the loved one is not so much the result of logical deduction as the inner evidence of friendship itself....In human friendship there is an archetypal proof that needs no further proof for human love—the presence of the friend, the opportunity of a limitless unfolding before him, and the presence of the Absolute which makes all this possible....Friendship makes clear the unshakable soul-shattering presence of absolute goodness.

It is in this death-defying component of love that playfulness takes its origin. If no evil power, however strong, can overcome love, then there is no reason not to play. The refusal to play is a hedging of the bet. We will love, yes, but we will keep some restrictions, some restraints and controls on that love as a hedge against the tragedy of its coming to an end. In a world dominated by evil, suffering, and death there is little about which to be playful. Play in such circumstances is childish, frivolous, and irresponsible. Ironic and sardonic laughter is permitted, but joyous merriment is foolish and self-deceptive. There is, after all, relatively little to laugh about if death simply means oblivion.

Obviously, most people do not think these things explicitly. I am talking not about a conscious process of thought and emotion that goes on in a sustained sexual relationship but about the psychological and existential dynamics through which people make their choices. The choice can be light or heavy, comic or tragic, hopeful or despairing. In a universe in which neither alternative of each pair is self-evident, the choice is rarely made in so many words. We make it, rather, by the way we live, by the little risks we do or do not take, the little opportunities we seize or do not seize, the little chances we grab as they float by or ignore without a second glance. The fundamental option that guides our life is made slowly and gradually. We see it forming a pattern for our life only when we look back. We do not simply exercise a fundamental option for or against laughter on any given day. It is the small choices, the drift as well as the decision, that determine that fundamental choice. We move from predisposition to fundamental option without being very clear about what we are doing. We discover our choice only when its inevitable long-term effects are so obvious that we can ignore them no longer.

Resentment, self-pity, the imposition of obligations on the other are characteristics of a nonplayful sexual relationship. We develop a long list of the things that the other has done and the burdens we have had to tolerate. We feel terribly sorry for all the things we had to put up with, and seek consolation from others who will agree (if only to escape) with us. The resentments rooted in self-pity are precious. They give meaning and purpose to our life; they organize the phenomena of experience. To lose them would be to lose an important part of the self. Yet we never make a decision to go down the path of self-pity and resentment; we simply know that when we are at the end of the path we discover that we have been walking on it for a long, long time.

We can make our relationships ones of formal exchange and barter. "I will do this if you will do that." We can even institutionalize these arrangements in formal marriage contracts, as some defiant, progressive young people do, and specify the obligations and responsibilities each partner will assume in the marriage. But the mutual-obligation approach to marriage need not be explicit or formal, and in most cases it is not. In fact, those who are locked into that style are frequently surprised when they are told that their marriage is nothing more than a system of mutual obligation. They never decided to make it that, and yet they surely and inevitably made a long series of decisions leading to a network of mutual obligations binding them in a constricted and inhibited relationship. There is no way that the light touch of playfulness, with its gratuitousness, its triviality, its spontaneity, its apparent foolishness, can loosen the bonds of mutual obligation. The essence of play is that one doesn't have to do it but decides on the spur of the moment to have some fun. When play is codified, regimented, regulated, defined, it stops being play. (I do not deny the insight of social theorists, like George Caspar Homans, Peter Blau, and Michael Hechter, who see intimacy as an exchange relationship. Exchange there surely is, but there must be something more besides. Even Homans and Blau stop short of viewing such exchange in terms of strict classical economics.)

The self-pity-resentment style and the obligation style are both familiar modalities of contemporary marriage. In these two modalities there is not room for playfulness. Indeed it is probably the case that most contemporary American marriages that are not playful stop short of it because they are caught in the self-pity or obligation or both styles of marriage. Thus do the powers death and despair constrain and restrict our fundamental life options without our ever having quite the insight to see how they are doing it.

Only when something catches us up short, only when some sort of dramatic event forces us to review the pattern of our life and to see the shape of our fundamental options do we see how far we have come and in what direction. Only in that revelation can we grasp the options we have chosen to exclude. It is for most of us not a pleasant experience.

But options can be modified and even changed. It is never too late to start over. Indeed, starting over is of the essence of life, and we are only truly dead when we have lost our capacity for beginning again. Every day is or can be a new beginning. No matter how long a relationship has lasted, no matter what direction it has moved in, no matter what fundamental options and their resultant styles have dominated our relationship, it is still possible to begin anew. It cannot be done without reference to what has gone before, but with relative freedom from its inevitability. One is never too old to grow, to change. It gets harder, but we can do it. Our relationships can begin to be playful even today, and if there is any life or vitality left at all, the spontaneous impulses that leap from love to playfulness can be revived. As long as we have not become so deadly serious (and that is to say, dead) that we cannot laugh at ourselves, then we can play. The first step in beginning to play is to laugh at oneself, or, to put it differently, when we resolve not to take ourself so damn seriously we have begun to break the constraints of resentment, self-pity, and obligation. After that anything can happen.

And there, of course, is the problem. What will happen when anything can happen? We have no way of knowing. Bad things as well as good things, perhaps. We maintain rigid control of our lives because we are afraid that if we don't something may happen—death may happen. To avoid that possibility we exclude the playfulness, the pleasure, the joy that may also occur when we open ourselves to the "anything-may-happen" situation.

Death will happen anyhow. The question is whether we will go through life in constant terror of it, or whether we can go through life laughing at it because we believe we will conquer that terror. If we are not willing to laugh at death and all its surrogates, then we will flee from beginning over again, starting anew, seizing the second chance.

Strangely enough, the experience of starting over again, of rediscovering one another, is one of such special delight that it is astonishing that a man or woman should consider it difficult. These delights are not available to those starting fresh. The mystery of discovery and the discovery of mystery are intensely more pleasurable when we share them with an old friend suddenly become new again.

But starting over seems to be painful for most.

One must give death to the illusions, deceptions, pretenses, and styles of relating that have become as natural as the air we breathe. We must give death to the illusion that we need not change, that we must fear change, and that we must fear to begin to change. It is indeed the fear of death that prevents us from beginning again, because beginning again is a form of death.

Hence the ultimate question: What comes after death? Annihilation? Something else? Or Some One else? Every new beginning is a death and resurrection. When a man and woman decide to restructure their relationship they are running a risk of encountering nothingness. It is truly dying. Yet they may discover someone, a lover with whom to play in sexual intimacy. For the Christian man and woman it is a foretaste, a hint of the Lover with whom we expect to play for all eternity.

Sexual play is a reflection of the playing of the Word and the Spirit that gave birth to the cosmos. It is an anticipation of the endless play of the life after resurrection. In the Christian world view sexual play is either both of those things or a monstrous deception. As Father Boros points out, once one is swept up by the game, one has no doubts. It is more real than anything else; it is the *realest* thing there is: It is an Anticipation of the Absolute.